Who Has the Cure?

Who Has the Cure?

Hamilton Project Ideas on Health Care

JASON FURMAN
editor

BROOKINGS INSTITUTION PRESS
Washington, D.C.

Library of Congress Cataloging-in-Publication data
Who has the cure? : Hamilton Project ideas on health care / Jason Furman, editor.
   p. cm.
  Includes bibliographical references and index.
  Summary: "Emphasizes the importance of universal health care and looks at
alternatives for achieving universal health care coverage that also improves
efficiency in the health care industry and provides proposals to improve the
effectiveness and affordability of health care, including income-related cost-
sharing, expanding preventive care, and reforming Medicare's prescription
benefit"—Provided by publisher.
  ISBN 978-0-8157-3008-8 (cloth : alk. paper) — ISBN 978-0-8157-3009-5
(pbk. : alk. paper) 1. Right to health care—United States. 2. Health services
accessibility—United States. 3. Health insurance—United States. 4. National
health insurance—United States. 5. Health care reform—United States.
I. Furman, Jason. II. Hamilton Project.
  [DNLM: 1. National Health Insurance, United States—United States.
2. Universal Coverage—United States. W 275 AA1 W476 2008]
  RA395.A3W488 2008
  362.10973—dc22   2008041974

9 8 7 6 5 4 3 2 1

Typeset in Sabon and Frutiger

Composition by Circle Graphics
Columbia, Maryland

Printed by R. R. Donnelley
Harrisonburg, Virginia

Contents

Acknowledgments

Over the past several years, many leading policy figures have shared their wisdom, advice, and insights with The Hamilton Project as we developed the economic strategy underlying our work and the specific policy proposals that promote that strategy. Though too many to name, we are grateful to all for their generosity, support, and unwavering insistence on analytical rigor. We are particularly grateful to The Hamilton Project's Advisory Council members, who have sustained and guided our efforts and without whom our policy work would not be possible. The Hamilton Project has been fortunate to attract an exceptionally talented cadre of staff members over the years who have helped bring our policy proposals to fruition, and we thank all of them for their inspired work and dedication to our mission. The Hamilton Project has also benefited enormously from making its home within one of the nation's most respected think tanks, and we are very grateful to the leadership and staff of the Brookings Institution for their continued support and encouragement. Finally, we wish to thank the many leading academics and analysts who shared their innovative ideas for policy reform with us and drew on their vast expertise and empirical research to develop those ideas into Hamilton Project discussion papers and subsequent chapters here.

Universal, Effective, and Affordable Health Insurance

An Economic Imperative

JASON FURMAN AND ROBERT E. RUBIN

T he Hamilton Project was founded to develop an economic strategy together with innovative policy ideas to promote three goals: growth, broad-based participation in growth, and economic security in a changing global economy. The Project's proposals span a wide range of policy areas including education, income security, health, science and technology, tax policy, climate change, energy security, workforce training, and poverty reduction. The proposals have come from leading academics, practitioners, and policy analysts from across the nation, taking cutting-edge and evidence-based ideas from economists and others and bringing them to bear on policy debates in a relevant, accessible, and actionable way. Each idea is offered as a potentially innovative step in the right direction to upgrade the country's policies, though they are not collectively a comprehensive "solution" to the nation's challenges. Rather, they are intended to provoke thought and discussion and serve as a portfolio of options from which policymakers may choose.

In a previous volume, The Hamilton Project collected its proposals in the areas of income security, education, and tax policy (Bordoff and Furman 2008). In this volume, we turn to another central element of an effective economic strategy: achieving universal health insurance coverage that is both affordable and effective. Access to health care is not just a major social objective but also an economic imperative.

In total 45 million Americans are uninsured, and the Institute of Medicine (2003) estimates that 18,000 of them die prematurely each year as a result. But the problems are much broader than just the uninsured. The typical insured family pays, directly and indirectly, more than one-sixth of its income for health care. And this expensive care is far less effective than it should be: Americans get too little preventive care when well, and only 55 percent of proven-effective therapies are administered when they are sick. At the same time, one-third or more of many major medical procedures are either inappropriate or of debatable value (McGlynn 1998; McGlynn and others 2003).

Moreover, the problems of uninsurance and expensive or ineffective care are interrelated. More medically effective care could also be more affordable, reducing the number of uninsured. Conversely, it is impossible to address fully the problems of affordability and effectiveness without covering everyone. Much of the health care the uninsured do get is costly and inefficient, with the costs passed on to others. Insuring everyone would not just eliminate these uncompensated cost shifts, it would also enable the health system to function better by expanding risk pooling and reducing the fragmentation of financing.

Responding to these interrelated health challenges is also critical for economic performance more broadly for four reasons:

—*Rapidly rising premiums put a strain on businesses, wages, and jobs.* When premiums jumped 52 percent from 2000 to 2005 (in inflation-adjusted terms), the rising cost of compensating workers led businesses to cut jobs, particularly in sectors like manufacturing that tend to offer workers good health coverage (Kaiser Family Foundation and Health Research and Educational Trust 2006; Reber and Tyson 2004). Over a longer period, workers generally bear the cost of higher premiums in the form of lower wages. Finally, rising premiums have led employers to drop coverage: the percentage of nonelderly Americans with employer-sponsored insurance has fallen from 70 percent in 1987 to 62 percent in 2005 (DeNavas-Walt, Proctor, and Lee 2006).

—*Ineffective care results in a less productive workforce* that misses more days of work and performs less effectively on the job. The benefits of better health care create a positive externality for other workers and other firms that is not captured by the individuals or employers paying for the health care, creating an important role for government in public health and other areas.

—*The rapid increase in public health spending is a central cause of the serious fiscal challenges* we face in the years and decades ahead, a challenge that represents a deep threat to our economic well-being if not addressed. Solving the long-run financing challenges facing Medicare and Medicaid requires addressing the similar growth in health spending taking place in the private sector.

—*Health care security is an important piece of the broader question of economic security.* America's patchwork, incomplete system of health insurance impedes the flexibility the economy needs to thrive and grow. Many workers are effectively locked into their jobs because they fear losing health insurance. According to one study, labor mobility is 25 percent less for those with employer-sponsored health insurance than for those without it (Madrian 1994). Moreover, the market-based economics and trade liberalization that are key to strong growth are more politically sustainable when workers have a greater sense of security and feel that they have more to gain and less to lose from the global economy.

In the chapters that follow in this book, leading experts offer innovative ideas about how a combination of private markets and effective government policies can reform health care. The next four chapters contain four alternative proposals to achieve universal health care coverage, and the following three chapters contain three proposals intended to promote greater affordability and more effectiveness in the health care system.

The proposals in this book represent the views of their authors and do not reflect a specific position taken by The Hamilton Project. In some cases the approaches are complementary; in other cases they represent alternatives to achieve the Project's broad goals of promoting growth, broad-based participation in growth, and economic security. In every case they are intended to be innovative ideas that will promote discussion and debate on one of the central economic challenges facing the United States.

Achieving Universal Coverage

Chapters 2 through 5 lay out four different approaches to achieving universal health care coverage. Although they all agree on the same goal of expanding access to health care, the proposals represent a wide range of philosophical approaches.

In chapter 2 Gerard Anderson and Hugh Waters of the Johns Hopkins Bloomberg School of Public Health propose expanding a well-known public health insurance program—Medicare—to offer an affordable coverage option to all firms and individuals wishing to buy into it. Instead of requiring fundamentally new ways of operating, their proposal for Medicare Part E(veryone) is guided by the principle that a practical universal coverage proposal should minimize disruptions and costs. Therefore, their proposal would allow individuals to keep their current employer-sponsored coverage while also offering insurance to all Americans through Medicare. Their proposal achieves universal coverage by requiring individuals to acquire health insurance (with federal subsidies for low-income households) and requiring firms to provide it. By building on the history and experience of Medicare, Anderson and Waters aim for a feasible plan that provides affordable, continuous, and efficient health care coverage to everyone.

Stuart Butler of the Heritage Foundation addresses in chapter 3 the growing mismatch between the current health insurance system, which works best for long-serving employees of large firms, and the realities of today's workforce, in which workers are increasingly mobile, part-time, self-employed, or employed by smaller firms. Butler's proposed reform calls for the creation of the Health Exchange Plan. Operating in parallel with—rather than replacing—the employer-sponsored system, the plan is designed to fill in the present system's gaps. Butler's plan contains three key steps that he argues are needed to achieve a gradual transformation in the health insurance system without disrupting the successful parts of the system. First, states should establish "insurance exchanges." Exchanges would offer an array of coverage options, and families could retain their chosen plan from workplace to workplace with the same tax benefits as those available for traditional employer-sponsored plans. Second, most employers should become facilitators, rather than sponsors, of coverage. While many large employers would continue to sponsor coverage, most employers would hand over sponsorship to an insurance exchange and focus on providing administrative support for their employees' insurance choices. Third, the federal government should reform the tax treatment of health insurance to focus the benefits on lower-income families. By partly delinking the availability and the subsidy of health coverage from the workplace, Butler's plan aims at evolutionary reform of the current system that would enhance economic and health security for all working families.

In chapter 4 Ezekiel Emanuel of the National Institutes of Health and Victor Fuchs of Stanford University propose a major health care reform to achieve universal and continuous coverage, control costs, and improve the quality of care. Under their proposed Guaranteed Health Care Access Plan, all Americans would receive a universal healthcare voucher to purchase a comprehensive benefit package through private insurance. The set of standard benefits would be modeled on a high-end plan currently available to federal employees. Private insurance firms would administer the program, and Americans would be able to choose their own physicians, hospitals, and health plans. The authors argue that their proposal would give private insurers more incentives to cut costs and compete on the basis of quality, and fewer incentives to discriminate against individuals based on their health since the government would pay insurers a risk-adjusted amount for each individual. The authors propose an independent National Health Board to define and adjust standard benefits, calculate premiums paid by the government, and sponsor research on quality and performance outcomes. The voucher system would establish an institute to evaluate the cost and effectiveness of drugs, medical devices, tests, and medical procedures, and another institute to resolve malpractice disputes. It would be funded through a dedicated value-added tax of 10 to 12 percent. Taking into account savings from administrative efficiency and the phasing out of public insurance, Emanuel and Fuchs argue that universal vouchers would be more effective and equitable than the current system without increasing total health care spending.

Finally, in chapter 5 Jonathan Gruber of the Massachusetts Institute of Technology examines the feasibility, costs, and benefits of extending nationwide the "Massachusetts model," which provides universal coverage through a combination of mandates, subsidies, and alternative insurance risk pools. Under Gruber's plan those happy with their current employer-sponsored health insurance plans could keep them, while those that want to change plans would have more affordable coverage choices than those available today. Like the Massachusetts model, which Gruber helped design, the national system would include subsidies for low-income Americans, pooling mechanisms to keep premiums low, and a requirement that all residents purchase health insurance. Gruber also proposes some important modifications to the Massachusetts model, however. His proposal would extend subsidies to households with incomes up to 400 percent of the federal poverty line to help middle-income families who do not have employer-based coverage. It would allow individuals with incomes below 400 percent of the poverty line who are not able to afford their employer's health insurance to use a voucher to buy health insurance in the low-income health insurance pool. And it would mandate insurance coverage for all individuals and improve enforcement of the mandate through the tax code. Modeling a national plan after the Massachusetts reforms, argues Gruber, would expand coverage and provide affordability to all Americans.

Enhancing Affordability and Effectiveness

To be successful, efforts to expand health insurance coverage must be coupled with efforts to make health care more affordable and effective. Chapters 6 through 8 target specific aspects of the system in which new policies could lower costs and improve the quality of care at the same time.

Richard Frank and Joseph Newhouse of Harvard University argue in chapter 6 that while the Medicare Part D prescription drug benefit provides welcome and important benefits, the program suffers from four significant limitations: a daunting complexity that has likely discouraged enrollment, incentives for insurance companies to avoid covering higher-cost individuals, inefficient purchasing rules that increase the cost of the program, and partial coverage (the so-called "doughnut hole") that leaves many seniors facing significant financial risks. In response, they propose four reforms. To reduce complexity, they would limit the number of prescription drug plans to between seven and nine and introduce automatic enrollment of seniors in a default drug plan, while preserving choice by allowing beneficiaries to change plans or to opt out entirely. To increase competition and reduce incentives to avoid serving high-cost seniors, they would require plan sponsors to compete for regional contracts rather than for individual enrollees. To enhance cost-effectiveness, they would adopt Medicaid's "best price" rule used for beneficiaries eligible for both Medicaid and Medicare, monitor the prices of unique drugs, and remove the distinction between Part D drugs and drugs still covered under Medicare Part B (which pays for outpatient services and has payment rules that differ from Part D, thus creating an opportunity for manufacturers to game the system to receive compensation from whichever part of Medicare will pay the most). Finally, to fill in the coverage gap, they would allow plans that are actuarially equivalent to the standard plan to offer higher deductibles in exchange for filling the doughnut hole.

Jason Furman of the Brookings Institution shows in chapter 7 that although families ultimately pay for all their health care costs, there has been a dramatic shift in the financing of health care over the past several decades away from out-of-pocket spending and toward insurance coverage. While more comprehensive health insurance benefits are largely a positive development, Furman offers empirical evidence that the increased insulation of consumers from direct out-of-pocket health care costs has also contributed to higher overall spending on health care, which, in turn, increases both the number of uninsured and the risks faced by those who have insurance. In response Furman advances a proposal for progressive cost sharing in health insurance. Furman rejects health savings account (HSA) approaches because they involve costly tax breaks for the affluent while increasing risks for low- and moderate-income families. Instead he suggests an alternative approach that bases cost sharing on income (limiting it to 7.5 percent of a family's income and even less for low- and moderate-income families) and potentially includes evidence-based exceptions for highly valuable treatments and preventive care. Furman estimates that progressive cost sharing could reduce health insurance premiums by 22 to 34 percent without compromising health outcomes. This approach provides robust protection against major risks, providing every family with an affordable ceiling on out-of-pocket spending. In addition, out-of-pocket expenses would fall for 23 percent of families, primarily low- and moderate-income families and families with large out-of-pocket expenses.

In chapter 8 Jeanne Lambrew of the Lyndon B. Johnson School of Public Affairs and the Center for American Progress proposes a Wellness Trust to prioritize disease prevention. Chronic and preventable diseases currently account for most costs, as well as deaths, in the health care system, despite the relatively low-cost and low-tech services that could limit them. Disease prevention and health promotion are crucial for ensuring the health and well-being of Americans in a cost-effective manner, but the current system is ill-suited to achieve these goals. People often are unaware of preventive services, perceive them as having low value, or are deterred by costs. Moreover, the myopic focus of the health care system on treating disease crowds out resources and directs incentives away from preventive care that fosters long-term wellness. Lambrew's Wellness Trust would be formed by carving preventive services out of disparate pieces of the health care system and uniting them under a single agency with the appropriate mission, incentives, and tools to deliver those services. The Wellness Trust would set national prevention priorities based on evidence of their impact, cost, and feasibility. It would employ effective delivery systems by connecting individuals to accessible and affordable preventive services, for example, through better communications and record-keeping, greater training of health care workers in preventive care, and state and local grants that incorporate prevention priorities. The Wellness Trust would also use payment incentives to encourage appropriate delivery, high standards, and greater take-up of preventive services. Finally, it would draw from public and private resources currently spent on prevention to fund its activities. By gearing the national health care system toward effective prevention, Lambrew's proposal could eventually lower insurance premiums and improve the quality of treatment, thereby contributing to a healthier and more productive nation.

Conclusion

The chapters in this book offer innovative and evidence-based proposals to inform the public policy debate over health care reform by laying out a promising path toward expanding health insurance coverage and increasing the affordability and effectiveness of health care in the United States. Achieving these objectives is among the most pressing economic policy issues facing our country. By meeting our nation's health care challenges, we can go a long way toward enhancing the economic security of individual workers, strengthening America's businesses as they struggle to compete in the global economy, and increasing our nation's overall productivity and fiscal soundness.

References

DeNavas-Walt, Carmen, Bernadette D. Proctor, and Cheryl Hill Lee. 2006. *Income, Poverty, and Health Insurance Coverage in the United States: 2005.* Current Population Reports P60-231. U.S. Census Bureau.

Institute of Medicine. 2003. *Hidden Costs, Value Lost: Uninsurance in America.* Consequences of Uninsurance series. Washington: National Academy of Sciences.

Furman, Jason, and Jason Bordoff, eds. 2008. *Path to Prosperity: Hamilton Project Ideas on Income Security, Education and Taxes.* Brookings.

Kaiser Family Foundation and Health Research and Educational Trust. 2006. *Employer Health Benefits 2006: Annual Survey.* Washington.

Madrian, Brigitte C. 1994. "Employment-Based Health Insurance and Job Mobility: Is There Evidence of Job-Lock?" *Quarterly Journal of Economics* 109, no. 1: 27–51.

McGlynn, Elizabeth A. 1998. "Assessing the Appropriateness of Care: How Much Is Too Much?" Research Brief RB-4522. Santa Monica, Calif.: RAND.

McGlynn, Elizabeth A., and others. 2003. "The Quality of Health Care Delivered to Adults in the United States." *New England Journal of Medicine* 348, no. 26: 2635–45.

Reber, Sarah, and Laura Tyson. 2004. "Rising Health Insurance Costs Slow Job Growth and Reduce Wages and Job Quality." Working Paper. Washington: Kaiser Family Foundation.

Achieving Universal Coverage through Medicare Part E(veryone)

2

GERARD F. ANDERSON AND HUGH R. WATERS

Our starting premise is that any proposal to provide universal health coverage should be simple to explain so that members of the public can assess how any changes would affect them personally. Medicare Part E(veryone) is designed to be easy for the public to understand: it builds on the existing Medicare system and makes minimal changes to the rest of the health care system. Although we developed Part E as a self-contained program, policymakers could choose to combine it with a more ambitious restructuring of the health care system.

Our proposal to add a Medicare Part E is simple: make the benefits that current Medicare beneficiaries receive available to everyone. This expansion achieves universal coverage using the existing Medicare rules and payment systems. Under our proposal, all individuals are required to have health insurance. Those with existing insurance coverage will not have to change to Medicare Part E unless they or their employers want to change,

Bianca Frogner, a doctoral student in health economics at Johns Hopkins, performed some of the analysis and participated in the drafting of the paper. The authors would like to thank her for her outstanding assistance. Karen Davis and Len Nichols carefully reviewed an earlier draft and made numerous helpful comments. Jason Bordoff, Jason Furman, Douglas Elmendorf, Sara Heller, and Brian Prest at the Hamilton Project improved the final version immensely.

as long as their public or private health insurance coverage meets certain minimum criteria. Firms will be able to buy into the Medicare Part E program, and individuals without employer-based coverage will be able to enroll on their own. In the case of firms participating in Part E, the employer will be required to pay at least as much of the premium as each employee, all of whom are required to enroll.

Part E is financed through a standard premium; everyone is charged the same amount. The federal government, however, provides a sliding-scale subsidy to help cover the cost of the premium for households whose income is below 400 percent of the federal poverty level (FPL). The level of the subsidy is based on the wage income of the household, where income is determined by how much the household pays in Medicare payroll tax. Premiums will be set so that the program breaks even, net of the subsidy.

Motivation for the Proposal

The structure of our Medicare Part E proposal is motivated by the Institute of Medicine's (IOM) recommended five guiding criteria for considering health insurance expansion options. The IOM's five criteria are universality, continuity, affordability for individuals and families, affordability and sustainability for society, and enhancement of the population's health status (IOM 2004). We believe, first, that universal health insurance coverage is necessary to improve the health status of Americans who are not currently covered or who have inadequate health insurance coverage. Several IOM studies have documented the benefits of insurance coverage (IOM 2001, 2002a, 2002b, 2003a, 2003b, 2004). Second, there should be no gaps in coverage when people change jobs, move, or fail to sign up for coverage. Third, the option providing adequate coverage at the least cost to individuals and to society should be chosen. Fourth, the private sector should be involved when it can add value. Fifth, the method for covering the uninsured should be easy to explain and should be built on the existing infrastructure so that it can be implemented quickly. Finally, although additional reforms to the health care system—including cost containment initiatives—are desirable, they should not be a prerequisite to universal coverage. Medicare Part E pursues these goals in the following ways.

Universality and Continuity

Individuals are mandated to purchase health insurance, employers are mandated to offer health insurance, and federal government subsidies are designed to make health insurance affordable to low-income individuals. By offering an accessible option outside of the employer-based health care system, Part E would reduce the medical and financial uncertainty that currently results from lapses in coverage when workers switch jobs or working arrangements.

Affordability

In implementing universal health insurance, it is important to ensure that the new option is affordable on both the societal and individual levels. We believe that the least expensive option on both counts is to offer Medicare coverage to the uninsured. Part E will have significantly lower administrative costs than an expansion of private insurance, and it is more appropriate than Medicaid for a variety of logistical and economic reasons outlined further on in this discussion. Part E would keep down the cost for individuals and firms, who would be required to purchase coverage, as well as for taxpayers, who would be required to subsidize the coverage of low-income individuals. We predict that Part E would be cheaper on an individual level, with premiums for a family of four dropping to $10,000 from the current average family premium of $11,480.

Added Value from the Private Sector

The private sector will be encouraged to participate when it has the ability to provide a better product at a lower or similar cost. Under our proposal, private insurance can be sold to individuals and employers, and these private health plans must meet only minimal requirements in order to qualify. In addition, private health plans are able to participate under Medicare Parts C and D, and are able to sell Medigap coverage.

Simplicity and Feasibility

Our plan adds a new option but, unlike many other universal coverage proposals, does not require changes to any of the existing options, including the employer-sponsored health insurance system, Medicaid, the State Children's Health Insurance Program (SCHIP), and Medicare for current beneficiaries. To this end, we maintain the existing tax exclusion for employer contributions to health insurance, both for private insurance plans and for employer contributions to the new Medicare Part E plans. By establishing universal coverage through the current system rather than in place of it, our proposal should be much more politically feasible than other reforms that affect many different constituencies.

Why Medicare?

The Medicare benefit package offers sufficient coverage for the uninsured without imposing excessive costs. However, we recognize that there are limitations to the Medicare benefit package, such as high levels of cost sharing, inadequate long-term care coverage, lack of transportation to medical services, and insufficient coverage for some chronic conditions. When the Medicare program was constructed in 1965, it was designed primarily for acute care, and now most of the utilization is for chronic care. We believe there are provisions in the Medicare program that should be changed. However, the Medicare program represents more than forty years of political compromises and has benefited from countless analytical studies. As a result, we have chosen not to modify the Medicare program.

We also recognize that some of the Medicare benefits may not be perfect for children, pregnant women, and younger adults. However, 15 percent of Medicare enrollees are disabled individuals who are under age sixty-five, and the benefit package covers their needs. For example, although Medicare's benefits may not be ideal for pregnant women, the current system already provides support when disabled women become pregnant. We anticipate that the Medicare program will continue to evolve and improve. Medicare Part E may actually accelerate this transformation because it will give Medicare additional market power.

We acknowledge that the Medicaid benefit package is more comprehensive and may be more appropriate for low-income individuals. If long-term care and other standard Medicaid benefits are included, then Medicaid is also more expensive than many other purely health insurance packages. Though there are studies that demonstrate that Medicaid is actually less expensive than private insurance on a comparable per person basis (Hadley and Holahan 2003–04; Miller, Banthin, and Moeller 2004), Medicaid's lesser expense stems primarily from lower payments to health care providers than those that private insurance (or Medicare) provides. As such, Medicaid is likely to be unpopular with providers and may be unable to attract a sufficient number of providers for a universal health plan. Additionally, because the Medicaid benefit package is more comprehensive than either Medicare or most private insurance benefit packages, an expansion of Medicaid is likely to be opposed by Medicare beneficiaries and people with private insurance wondering why they do not receive such a comprehensive benefit package. For these reasons, we have not chosen the Medicaid benefit package. We assume no changes in the current Medicaid program.

Who Is Covered?

In developing the model and the cost estimates, we make several assumptions to calculate the number of people who would enroll in a new Part E. We assume that the number of uninsured adults in the United States will continue to increase at current rates in the absence of reform. Approximately 1 million adults are added to the ranks of the uninsured every year (Kaiser Commission on Medicaid and the Uninsured 2006b). Currently, it is estimated that 8 million children do not have health insurance coverage (Holahan, Cook, and Dubay 2007). We assume that SCHIP will cover all of the low-income children it currently does; Part E will cover the 6.5 million children currently eligible for SCHIP but not enrolled. According to studies, only 4 percent of children above 300 percent of the FPL are uninsured (Dubay, Holahan, and Cook 2007). Nonetheless, we assume most families in this income range would seek to keep their children under the same policy as the adults, and we adjust take-up rates accordingly.

Additionally, our proposed Medicare Part E would cover undocumented immigrants who pay Medicare payroll taxes. Any undocumented immigrants who do not pay their taxes would not be covered under our plan and would need to continue to receive care from public clinics and private sources.

Medicare Part E

Flat premiums would be the primary financing mechanism for Medicare Part E. The value of the premium will reflect the actuarial value of the coverage, as calculated by Medicare actuaries. The premium will be split among employers, employees, and the federal government. Higher-income beneficiaries—those with incomes above 400 percent of the FPL, or about $80,000 for a family of four in 2006—would share a premium reflecting the full cost of the insurance with their employers, while lower-income beneficiaries would receive a sliding-scale subsidy paid through government general revenues.[1] In addition, workers and employers would continue to pay the 2.9 percent payroll tax that funds the current Medicare Part A program, and individuals who qualify for Medicare under current law would continue to pay premiums under current rules. This financing mechanism is

---

1. The FPL is commonly used for federal means-tested programs. In 2007 the poverty threshold cited by the Department of Health and Human Services for a family of four living in the forty-eight contiguous states and Washington, D.C., was $20,650.

designed to be both sustainable and fair. The value of the premium is adjusted every year to reflect changes in the cost of the program.

Household income as a percentage of the FPL will be determined through the income tax system. We use this measure of income because the FPL takes into account the size and earnings of the entire household. We acknowledge, however, that it may be administratively difficult to communicate to employers each employee's FPL on a timely basis, which is important because it affects what both the employer and employee pay. Should the administrative problems prove too difficult, alternatives could be considered, such as a flat tax rate based solely on wage income during the pay period.

A review of the existing proposals to cover the uninsured shows that most proposals base the subsidy on the FPL, and 400 percent of the FPL is the most common threshold. In Medicare Part E, persons whose Medicare income is above 400 percent of the FPL would not receive a federal subsidy. The formula for calculating the share of the Medicare Part E premium to be contributed by government (the subsidy) is 1 − (percent FPL)/400. The continuous formula prevents discontinuities in coverage by income. The formula for calculating the share of the Part E contribution to be contributed by the employer (if any) and the individual is (percent FPL/400). If there is no employer, then the employer's share would be covered by the individual, as under current Medicare law. Under this proposal, each person would be expected to contribute something to his or her insurance coverage and to the coverage of any dependents that do not qualify to receive other government-sponsored health insurance (such as SCHIP). People would be expected to purchase individual coverage in Medicare Part E.

Table 2-1 illustrates the percentage of the Part E premium that will be paid by the government, the individual, and the employer at various levels of the FPL. Although this payment structure explains the theory behind Part E funding, actual payment distributions may differ somewhat from what is listed here (see discussion in section on cost estimates).

As is true in the current Medicare program, the premium would be nationally rated (not risk adjusted), and there would be no geographic adjustments for the cost of medical care in the area where each individual lives. As stated above, the premium will be calculated based on the actuarial value of the package, adjusted by Medicare actuaries based on the previous year's experience. Because of its open enrollment and flat premium, and because the implementation of Medicare Part E will be accompanied by an insurance mandate, it is quite likely that the program will experience adverse risk selection in the sense that relatively unhealthy individuals will

Table 2-1. Employer, Individual, and Government Contributions to Medicare Part E Premiums

Percent

Percent of federal poverty level	Contribution		
	Employer	Individual	Government
0–50	0	0	100
51–100	6.25	6.25	87.5
101–200	12.5	12.5	75
201–300	25	25	50
301–400	37.5	37.5	25
401+	50	50	0

Source: Authors' calculations.

join it and relatively healthy individuals will seek lower-cost insurance options in the private sector.

To counteract this adverse selection and to ensure the fiscal solvency of Medicare Part E, the proposal could be adapted so that the federal government provides a subsidy to the program equivalent to the actuarial value of the risk adjustment each year—in other words, the financial value of the difference between the average actuarial value of the benefits package for the full under-sixty-five U.S. population and the actuarial value of the same package when offered to the Medicare Part E population. This adaptation would ensure that the share of the premium paid by firms and individuals would remain affordable. This is a policy that would by itself discourage, to some extent, the adverse selection that the program is likely to encounter. However, since the extent of adverse selection and its effect on Part E premiums are impossible to predict and would need to be monitored on an annual basis, we leave government subsidies of risk selection to the Medicare actuaries to monitor.

The objective in setting the premium rate is to make the Medicare Part E program financially self-sustaining, after taking account of the income-related subsidies that will be financed from general government revenues. Of course, there will be year-to-year fluctuations because of problems with actuarial projections and unexpected circumstances. As a result, the Part E program will have a small surplus in some years to be offset by small deficits in other years. No long-term deficits or surpluses are permitted.

The payment system under Part E would be the same as the Medicare program and would be updated as the Medicare program changes. The advantage of this approach is the clearly specified payment rules under the current Medicare program. All Medicare provisions would apply to Medicare Part E. The additional bureaucracy necessary to administer the program would be minimal because the current Medicare rules and regulations would apply. The Medicare collection mechanisms are already in place.

It is usually difficult to anticipate all the responses when new programs are implemented. It would be relatively easy to predict the responses of the various actors under Medicare Part E since the Medicare program has existed for more than forty years and is continuously monitored.

Benefits Included in Medicare Part E

The benefit package remains the same as under the Medicare program. Part E participants would have access to Parts A, B, C, and D since the Medicare Part E program would use the existing Medicare rules and regulations. Medicare Part E enrollees would also be permitted to purchase Medigap coverage under the same rules as current Medicare beneficiaries. Medigap premiums would not have income-related subsidies.

We expect that Medicare Parts A to D will continue to evolve and foster the adoption of quality-of-care initiatives (such as coordinated care for patients with chronic conditions) and to provide incentives to providers to adopt new technologies (such as health information technology). Also, we anticipate that Medicare will adopt cost containment strategies to resolve sustainability issues for Parts A to D. Assessment of clinical effectiveness is an important component of Medicare modernization. Since enrollees under Medicare Part E have access to Parts A to D, enrollees are assumed to reap all the benefits of any changes made to the Medicare program.

Opting Out of Medicare Part E

Public or private coverage would need to meet only minimal standards in order to be deemed acceptable and to exempt the person from mandatory Part E enrollment. The only criterion is that the health plan or the insured person would be expected to pay the medical bill. Under Part E, if 98 percent of the medical bills for hospital and doctor services were paid by either the insurer or the patient, then the health plan would be considered acceptable. This rule allows the private sector maximum flexibility. If less than 98 percent of hospital and doctor bills were paid by either the patient or the insurer, the health plan would lose its accreditation status. Initially all health plans would qualify. Public insurance programs would qualify (for example, Medicaid), whereas public programs that simply provided services (community health centers, Veterans Health Administration, and so on) would not. People unable to pay their medical bills would be automatically enrolled in Medicare Part E for a five-year period unless they qualify for public insurance.

Allowing Individuals and Firms to Buy into Medicare Part E

In addition to the uninsured, everyone would be eligible to enroll in Medicare Part E. For individuals, small firms, larger firms with high-risk individuals, and larger firms with an older workforce, the Medicare Part E premium would probably be less expensive than the premium being offered in the marketplace. One reason for that cost difference is that plans offered through Medicare would have lower administrative costs. Moreover, a majority of the population would be eligible for subsidies if they purchased insurance through Medicare Part E.[2] This would create a major incentive for employers to switch to coverage through Medicare Part E.

If firms choose to enroll in Medicare Part E, they would be required to enroll all employees. Firms would not be permitted to enroll only high-risk individuals or only low-wage individuals. Calculations of the amounts to be paid by the individual, the employer, and the federal government would be based on the individual's income. As a result, firms with a high proportion of low-wage workers would get a larger subsidy from the federal government than would firms with higher-wage workers.

As an example, consider an individual making 100 percent of the FPL. She and her employer would each pay 12.5 percent of the premium (the amount expected at 100 percent FPL). The federal government would cover the remaining 75 percent. Firms that voluntarily decided to use the Medicare Part E program for health insurance coverage would need to remain in the Part E program for a minimum of two years. Firms with a high proportion of unhealthy workers may find Part E attractive, given the lower premiums than in the private sector. The federal government could also contribute a general revenue subsidy to account for possible adverse risk selection (see above).

2. U.S. Bureau of Labor Statistics and U.S. Census Bureau, "Current Population Survey (CPS) Table Creator for the Annual Social and Economic Supplement," 2006 (www.census. gov/hhes/www/cpstc/cps_table_creator.html).

Table 2-2. Administrative Costs of Medicare and Private Health Insurance, 2003

Dollars

Program	Administrative costs per beneficiary
Medicare[a]	137
Private health insurance	421

Sources: Kaiser Family Foundation, "Trends and Indicators in the Changing Health Care Marketplace," exhibit 6.11, April 11, 2005 (www.kff.org/insurance/7031/index.cfm); Hoffman, Klees, and Curtis (2004).

a. The Medicare administrative costs are an upper bound amount assuming that administrative costs are 2 percent of Medicare costs. However, the source estimates that administrative costs were less than 2 percent of the total Medicare costs.

Rationale for Expanding Medicare

Why Public Provision Is Less Expensive than Private Provision of Health Insurance

Since the federal government will be providing the subsidy for low-income workers, the federal government should choose the least expensive option to cover the uninsured. Public insurance programs are less expensive than private insurance in terms of administrative costs. Also called the loss ratio, this figure measures the amount that insurance companies retain and do not pay out in benefits. Administrative costs for a private health insurance beneficiary are more than three times the costs for a Medicare beneficiary (table 2-2). In addition, administrative costs are growing twice as fast among private insurers compared to the Medicare program. Between 1986 and 2003, administrative costs rose 400 percent for private insurers and 200 percent for Medicare.[3]

Administrative costs, however, might tell only a portion of the story: it is possible that higher administrative costs will actually lower total health care spending if private insurers are identifying ways both to eliminate fraud and abuse and to improve the efficiency of the delivery system. To examine this point, figure 2-1 compares the rates of increase in health care spending per capita in the Medicare and private health insurance programs from 1970 to 2004. In some years, the private sector was able to control health spending per capita more effectively than did the public sector, while in other years the reverse was true. Between 1970 and 2004, the annual rates of increase of spending per capita in the Medicare program were

3. Based on data from Centers for Medicare and Medicaid Services (CMS), "National Health Care Expenditures Data, Historical" (www.cms.hhs.gov/NationalHealthExpendData/02_NationalHealthAccountsHistorical.asp#TopOfPage), as well as unpublished CMS data on private health insurance enrollment.

Figure 2-1. Per Enrollee Growth in Medicare Spending and Private Health Insurance Premiums (for Common Benefits), 1970–2004

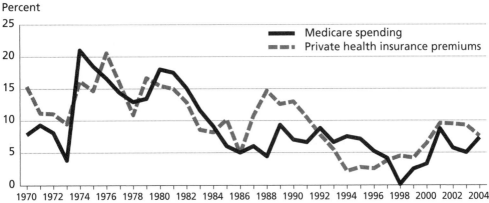

Source: CMS, "National Health Care Expenditures Data, Historical," table 13 (www.cms.hhs.gov/NationalHealthExpendData/02_NationalHealthAccountsHistorical.asp#TopOfPage).

lower than in the private sector—9.0 percent in the Medicare program compared to 10.1 percent in the private sector. This suggests that over the long run, the Medicare program has been more successful than the private insurance sector in controlling health care spending, in spite of the higher and growing administrative spending by private insurers.

Some have argued that managed care is clearly preferable to fee-for-service care. The Medicare program is predominately fee-for-service while the private sector is predominately managed care. Miller and Luft (1994, 1997, 2002) periodically evaluated the literature on the performance of fee-for-service and managed care, and at each review, the results suggested that the managed care plans were only marginally more successful than the fee-for-service plans at controlling aggregate spending. These literature reviews were published during the pinnacle of managed care in the mid- to late 1990s and early 2000s.

Since the last study published by Miller and Luft in 2002, the ability of managed care to control spending has diminished considerably, primarily because most consumers do not want to be presented with a restricted set of providers. As a result, the bargaining power of the managed care plans with doctors and hospitals has deteriorated (Blendon and others 2006). Data suggest that private sector insurance rates increased rapidly once consumers stopped accepting restrictions in their delivery network (Claxton and others 2006). Between 2000 and 2005, health insurance premiums increased an average of 11 percent per year. During this same time period, Medicare spending increased an average of 8.8 percent per year.

A recent comparison of the cost to the Medicare program of beneficiaries enrolled in fee-for-service versus managed care suggests that the higher administrative cost in the private sector may not provide additional benefits in terms of lower health care spending, and that beneficiaries enrolled in Part C may actually be more expensive for Medicare (Biles and others 2006). In our proposal, any additional subsidies to health plans in Medicare Part C would be eliminated.

Risk Selection in Private Insurance Interferes with Universality

A key objective of enrolling the uninsured is to achieve universality. Private health insurers have historically engaged in a variety of methods to achieve favorable selection. It is well known that a small proportion of the population accounts for a large portion of health care spending. This creates strong financial incentives for private insurers to engage in risk selection unless the payment system adjusts for the higher expected costs arising from these individuals. These are disproportionately individuals with chronic conditions. Therefore, it is likely that some private insurers will make it more difficult for uninsured persons with chronic conditions to obtain and retain health insurance coverage.

While it is possible to create legislation and regulations that prohibit certain actions by private health plans and to mandate provisions such as open enrollment and guaranteed renewal, the cost variations will still be a powerful incentive for private health plans to devise strategies that are one or two steps ahead of the rules and regulations. In contrast, the public sector does not have the profit motive and does not engage in competitive behavior. Therefore, risk selection is less likely to occur in the public sector. As a result, Medicare Part E will have fewer risk selection problems because of its reliance on community rating and guaranteed issue.

Medicare Part E Will Maintain Private Sector Involvement

There will be numerous opportunities for the private sector to participate in Medicare Part E, which in turn will be able to take advantage of the private sector's innovations under Medicare Parts C and D. Medicare beneficiaries are currently able to enroll in managed care options under Medicare Part C. The most innovative private sector options will be able to attract Medicare beneficiaries under Medicare Part C. Many private insurers participate in Medicare Part D. Private insurers will also be able to provide

Medigap coverage under Part E. We expect that the uninsured and individuals opting into Medicare Part E will be more likely to choose these options. In addition, health plans will still be able to provide private health insurance coverage as long as they meet minimal requirements.

Cost Estimates for Medicare Part E

Data Sources

In order to model the cost of Medicare Part E, we conducted a review of the literature concerning participation rates, crowd-out rates, the effects of premiums and copays on use, and the costs of coverage. We also reviewed the costs related to not having insurance. In addition to results from the literature, we use two principal data sources. The first is the March 2006 Current Population Survey (CPS) to measure current population insurance status and population characteristics.[4] The second is the Medical Expenditure Panel Survey (MEPS) for health expenditures for individuals with different self-perceived health status, differentiated by insurance status, income, and employment status.[5]

Steps in the Modeling Process

1. TAKE-UP FOR THOSE PREVIOUSLY UNINSURED (PARTICIPATION). We use the 2006 CPS and the 2004 MEPS to establish baseline estimates of the numbers of full-year uninsured individuals in the United States (tables 2-3 and 2-4). We calculate the number of individuals between the ages of eighteen and sixty-four in table 2-3 and children below the age of eighteen in table 2-4. We also summarize certain characteristics such as employment status, health status, and income level. Individuals older than sixty-four are assumed to have coverage under the existing Medicare insurance system.

Take-up rates refer to the percentage of individuals who will accept a new insurance coverage offer when it is presented to them. In the literature, predicted take-up rates for public insurance programs increase with individuals' age, educational status, and income. The rate for public insurance take-up most commonly used in studies for population groups below 150 percent of the FPL is 55 to 60 percent (Glied, Remler, and Zivin 2002). Because the implementation of Medicare Part E involves a mandate

4. U.S. Bureau of Labor Statistics and U.S. Census Bureau, "Current Population Survey," March 2006 (www.census.gov/cps/).

5. U.S. Department of Health and Human Services, Agency for Healthcare Research and Quality, "Medical Expenditure Panel Survey (MEPS)," 2004 (www.meps.ahrq.gov/mepsweb).

Table 2-3. Number of Uninsured Adults Ages Eighteen to Sixty-Four, by Income Level, Health Status, and Employment Status[a]

Employment and self-perceived health status	Income, by percent of FPL				
	<100	100–199	200–399	400+	Totals
Employed					
Excellent or good health	3,520,848	6,510,891	7,400,706	4,286,921	21,719,367
Poor or fair health	519,199	735,051	862,531	422,819	2,539,599
Unemployed					
Excellent or good health	609,280	578,593	650,707	298,915	2,137,495
Poor or fair health	250,588	173,563	112,553	50,416	587,120
Not in labor force					
Excellent or good health	2,915,381	2,102,708	1,658,991	797,928	7,475,008
Poor or fair health	1,582,174	1,141,138	900,332	433,035	4,056,679
Total uninsured adults	9,397,470	11,241,944	11,585,820	6,290,034	38,515,268
Excellent or good health	7,045,509	9,192,193	9,710,403	5,383,765	31,331,870
Poor or fair health	2,351,961	2,049,751	1,875,417	906,269	7,183,398

Source: Authors' calculations based on U.S. Bureau of Labor Statistics and U.S. Census Bureau, "Current Population Survey," March 2006 (www.census.gov/cps/).

a. Numbers may not sum to totals due to rounding.

for coverage, we assume these take-up rates will be higher than previous estimates.

We assume unemployed individuals will join at a 100 percent rate, since they will be unable to obtain insurance coverage through an employer and will find Medicare Part E considerably less expensive than private insurance options in the individual market. Conversely, higher-income individuals are predicted to participate at lower rates because they will be more likely to obtain insurance through an employer or in the individual market (table 2-5). To partly account for adverse selection and actions by private insurers, take-up rates are estimated to be higher for adults who have fair or poor self-reported health status.

Table 2-4. Number of Uninsured versus Insured under the Age of Eighteen, by Income Level[a]

Children under age eighteen	Income, by percent of FPL		
	<300	300+	Totals
Currently uninsured	6,527,233	1,367,413	7,894,647
Currently insured	35,349,205	30,041,256	65,390,461
Totals	41,876,439	31,408,669	73,285,108

Source: See table 2-3.

a. Numbers may not sum to totals due to rounding.

Table 2-5. Take-Up Rates for Uninsured Adults Ages Eighteen to Sixty-Four, by Income Level, Health Status, and Employment Status

Percent

Employment and self-perceived health status	Income, by percent of FPL			
	<100	100–199	200–399	400+
Employed				
Excellent or good health	60	55	40	25
Poor or fair health	85	80	65	50
Unemployed				
Excellent or good health	100	100	100	100
Poor or fair health	100	100	100	100
Not in labor force				
Excellent or good health	100	100	100	100
Poor or fair health	100	100	100	100

Source: Authors' estimations based on relevant literature.

Applying these percentages to the baseline numbers for uninsured adults from table 2-3 yields the total numbers of previously uninsured individuals who are predicted to join Medicare Part E (table 2-6).

2. TAKE-UP FOR THOSE WITH PREVIOUS PRIVATE INSURANCE (CROWD-OUT). Crowd-out refers to take-up into a public program by those who are already insured by another insurance plan. The crowd-out rate is typically defined as the percentage of individuals with private insurance who are eligible for a public program and who actually switch to the public program. For the purposes of Medicare Part E, we define crowd-out as the enrollment of individuals with any type of previous insurance—public or private—in Medicare Part E. We assume individuals that switch decide that Part E is the better and more affordable option. Table 2-7 shows the number of individuals aged eighteen to sixty-four in the United States who currently have insurance, broken down by income level, health status, and employment status.

As crowd-out rates increase, the efficiency of public insurance—comparing costs to the net increase in coverage—decreases. Estimates from the literature suggest that for the privately insured, the short-run elasticity (responsiveness) of take-up to a new program offer is approximately 30 percent as high as the elasticity of take-up among the uninsured (Glied, Remler, and Zivin 2002). Medicare Part E is likely to see higher crowd-out rates given the subsidization of the premium provided by the federal government. The subsidies will be particularly attractive for individuals with low to moderate levels of income. Firms would need to decide to opt

Table 2-6. Total Take-Up for Previously Uninsured Adults Ages Eighteen to Sixty-Four[a]

Number participating

Employment and self-perceived health status	Income, by percent of FPL				Totals
	<100	100–199	200–399	400+	
Employed					
Excellent or good health	2,112,509	3,580,990	2,960,282	1,071,730	9,725,512
Poor or fair health	441,319	588,040	560,645	211,409	1,801,414
Unemployed					
Excellent or good health	609,280	578,593	650,707	298,915	2,137,495
Poor or fair health	250,588	173,563	112,553	50,416	587,120
Not in labor force					
Excellent or good health	2,915,381	2,102,708	1,658,991	797,928	7,475,008
Poor or fair health	1,582,174	1,141,138	900,332	433,035	4,056,679
Total	7,911,251	8,165,033	6,843,511	2,863,434	25,783,228
Excellent or good health	5,637,170	6,262,292	5,269,980	2,168,574	19,338,015
Poor or fair health	2,274,081	1,902,741	1,573,531	694,860	6,445,213

Source: Authors' calculations based on tables 2-3 and 2-5.
a. Numbers may not sum to totals due to rounding.

Table 2-7. Number of Insured Adults Ages Eighteen to Sixty-Four, by Income Level, Health Status, and Employment Status

Employment and self-perceived health status	Income, by percent of FPL				Totals
	<100	100–199	200–399	400+	
Employed					
Excellent or good health	4,266,858	11,988,811	37,384,101	58,395,899	112,035,669
Poor or fair health	767,720	1,662,764	2,941,755	3,310,782	8,683,021
Unemployed					
Excellent or good health	4,360,641	3,207,886	5,563,340	6,915,970	20,047,837
Poor or fair health	2,969,509	1,854,218	1,778,550	1,239,885	7,842,162
Not in labor force					
Excellent or good health	21,765	23,055	121,232	121,203	287,255
Poor or fair health	4,013	5,061	21,477	6,990	37,541
Total insured adults	12,390,506	18,741,795	47,810,455	69,990,729	148,933,485
Excellent or good health	8,649,264	15,219,752	43,068,673	65,433,072	132,370,761
Poor or fair health	3,741,242	3,522,043	4,741,782	4,557,657	16,562,724

Source: Authors' calculations based on U.S. Bureau of Labor Statistics and U.S. Census Bureau, "Current Population Survey," March 2006 (www.census.gov/cps/) and on U.S. Department of Health and Human Services, Agency for Healthcare Research and Quality, "Medical Expenditure Panel Survey (MEPS)," 2004 (www.meps.ahrq.gov/mepsweb).

Table 2-8. Take-Up Rates for Previously Insured Adults (Crowd-Out) Ages Eighteen to Sixty-Four

Percent

Employment status	Income, by percent of FPL			
	<100	100–199	200–399	400+
Employed	65	60	55	50
Unemployed	30	25	22	20
Not in labor force	30	25	22	20

Source: Authors' estimations based on relevant literature.

in completely to Medicare Part E or to stay out of it completely: they cannot choose to place only some of their employees in the program. As a result, we predict the short-term effects of crowd-out into Medicare Part E to be as shown in tables 2-8 and 2-9. We expect crowd-out rates will increase over time as individuals and firms realize the value of Part E.

3. TOTAL ENROLLMENT IN MEDICARE PART E. Total adult enrollment (table 2-10) is a combination of participation (table 2-6) and crowd-out (table 2-9). Additionally, we predict that 24.3 million children below age eighteen would enroll in Part E from the following groups: approximately 6.5 million currently uninsured children that live in families below 300 percent of the FPL, and 17.8 million currently insured children

Table 2-9. Total Enrollment for Previously Insured Adults (Crowd-Out) Ages Eighteen to Sixty-Four[a]

Number enrolled

Employment and self-perceived health status	Income, by percent of FPL				Totals
	<100	100–199	200–399	400+	
Employed					
Excellent or good health	2,773,458	7,193,287	20,561,256	29,197,950	59,725,949
Poor or fair health	499,018	997,658	1,617,965	1,655,391	4,770,033
Unemployed					
Excellent or good health	1,308,192	801,972	1,223,935	1,383,194	4,717,293
Poor or fair health	890,853	463,555	391,281	247,977	1,993,665
Not in labor force					
Excellent or good health	6,530	5,764	26,671	24,241	63,205
Poor or fair health	1,204	1,265	4,725	1,398	8,592
Total	5,479,254	9,463,500	23,825,833	32,510,150	71,278,737
Excellent or good health	4,088,180	8,001,022	21,811,861	30,605,384	64,506,447
Poor or fair health	1,391,075	1,462,478	2,013,971	1,904,766	6,772,290

Source: Authors' calculations based on tables 2-7 and 2-8.
a. Numbers may not sum to totals due to rounding.

Table 2-10. Total Adult Enrollees, Ages Eighteen to Sixty-Four, in Medicare Part E[a]

Number enrolled

Employment and self-perceived health status	Income, by percent of FPL				Totals
	<100	100–199	200–399	400+	
Employed					
Excellent or good health	4,885,966	10,774,277	23,521,538	30,269,680	69,451,461
Poor or fair health	940,337	1,585,699	2,178,610	1,866,800	6,571,447
Unemployed					
Excellent or good health	1,917,472	1,380,565	1,874,642	1,682,109	6,854,788
Poor or fair health	1,141,441	637,117	503,834	298,393	2,580,785
Not in labor force					
Excellent or good health	2,921,910	2,108,472	1,685,662	822,169	7,538,213
Poor or fair health	1,583,378	1,142,403	905,057	434,433	4,065,271
Total adult enrollees	13,390,505	17,628,533	30,669,343	35,373,584	97,061,965
Excellent or good health	9,725,349	14,263,314	27,081,841	32,773,958	83,844,462
Poor or fair health	3,665,156	3,365,219	3,587,502	2,599,626	13,217,503

Source: Authors' calculations based on U.S. Bureau of Labor Statistics and U.S. Census Bureau, "Current Population Survey," March 2006 (www.census.gov/cps/).

a. Numbers may not sum to totals due to rounding.

from families above 300 percent of the FPL. This latter category is calculated based on crowd-out rates of 55 to 60 percent of the 30 million children above 300 percent of the FPL, assuming that most families in this income range would seek to keep their children under the same policy as the adults, whether that policy is private insurance or Medicare Part E.

4. EXPENDITURES. We base the estimates of expenditures under Medicare Part E on the 2004 MEPS, calculating current health expenditures for different health status groups by insurance status, income, and employment status (table 2-11). Accordingly, we project that the total annual

Table 2-11. Predicted Expenditures per Adult Enrollee, by Income Level and Health Status

Dollars

Health status	Income, by percent of FPL			
	<100	100–199	200–399	400+
Excellent or good health	4,413	4,483	4,574	4,458
Poor or fair health	6,468	6,273	6,192	5,937
Weighted average	4,975	4,825	4,763	4,567

Source: Authors' calculations based on U.S. Department of Health and Human Services, Agency for Healthcare Research and Quality, "Medical Expenditure Panel Survey (MEPS)," 2004 (www.meps.ahrq.gov/mepsweb).

Table 2-12. Total Predicted Expenditures for Adult Enrollees, by Income Level, Health Status, and Employment Status[a]

Billions of dollars

Employment and self-perceived health status	Income, by percent of FPL				
	<100	100–199	200–399	400+	Totals
Employed					
Excellent or good health	21.6	48.3	107.6	135.0	312.4
Poor or fair health	6.1	9.9	13.5	11.1	40.6
Unemployed					
Excellent or good health	8.5	6.2	8.6	7.5	30.7
Poor or fair health	7.4	4.0	3.1	1.8	16.3
Not in labor force					
Excellent or good health	12.9	9.5	7.7	3.7	33.7
Poor or fair health	10.2	7.2	5.6	2.6	25.6
Total expenditures, by health status					
Excellent or good health	42.9	63.9	123.9	146.1	376.8
Poor or fair health	23.7	21.1	22.2	15.4	82.5
Total predicted expenditures	...	...	...	...	459.3

Source: Authors' calculations based on U.S. Bureau of Labor Statistics and U.S. Census Bureau, "Current Population Survey," March 2006 (www.census.gov/cps/) and U.S. Department of Health and Human Services, Agency for Healthcare Research and Quality, "Medical Expenditure Panel Survey (MEPS)," 2004 (www.meps.ahrq.gov/mepsweb).

a. Numbers may not sum to totals due to rounding.

expenditures for adults in Medicare Part E will be $459.3 billion, adjusting for health status (table 2-12).

In addition, Medicare Part E will insure an estimated 24.3 million children under the age of eighteen, as calculated above. We estimate average annual expenditures for this age group of $1,200 per person, based on current Medicaid expenditures for this age group. As a result, Medicare Part E will have $29.1 billion in expenditures for children under age eighteen, for an overall total of $488.4 billion in expenditures. Of this amount, an estimated $60.2 billion will be paid through patient cost sharing—deductibles and copayments—for a net health care cost of $428.2 billion.

5. ADMINISTRATIVE COSTS. In addition to these expenditures, Medicare Part E will have administrative costs. Medicare's administrative costs are currently among the lowest of any insurer—public or private—in the United States. Average administrative costs per capita for Medicare are estimated to be $137, compared to $421 for private insurance.[6] Medicare

6. CMS, "National Health Expenditures by Type of Service and Source of Funds: Calendar Years 1960–2005" (www.cms.hhs.gov/NationalHealthExpendData/downloads/nhe2005.zip).

Part E will insure a total of 121.4 million beneficiaries—97.1 million adults and 24.3 million children. The resulting administrative costs will be $16.6 billion.

As a result, the combined annual health care costs and administrative costs for Medicare Part E are $444.8 billion. This is on the higher end of program cost ranges compared to other proposals (Collins, Davis, and Kriss 2007; Sheils and Haught 2003). However, all of the uninsured population will be covered under our proposal, and high-risk individuals will be subsidized.

6. CALCULATION OF THE PREMIUM. A guiding principle of Medicare Part E is that premiums are nationally rated; the same premium is charged to every adult enrollee (with subsidies based on income). In calculating the premium, we take into account the current Medicare cost-sharing arrangements—including a deductible for hospitalization, 20 percent copayments under Part B, and the existing cost-sharing structure for the pharmaceutical benefit. As a result, we calculate a total premium of $3,900 for adults and $1,100 for children; so a family of four would have an annual premium of $10,000 under Medicare Part E. In comparison, the average annual family premium for all Americans was $11,480 in 2006, and the average individual premium was $4,242.

The government's share of the Medicare Part E premium equals 1 − (percent FPL)/400; therefore, the share of the Part E premium to be contributed by the individual and employer (if any) is (percent FPL)/400. We start with the objective of splitting this part of the premium equally between employees and employers, with the federal government subsidizing each low-income worker. However, it is infeasible for the government to calculate separately the percent of the FPL for each employee in a firm. Therefore, our proposal would base government subsidies to each firm on the average wage at that firm. As a result, firms with a large proportion of high-income workers will receive a lower federal subsidy, since their average wage will be higher.

Workers above 400 percent of the FPL will still pay half of their premiums, and their employers will pay the other half. Workers below 400 percent of the FPL will pay a share of the premium equal to 1/2 (percent FPL)/400, and their employers will pay the remainder. Thus employers will pay as much as their workers in all cases and more than their workers in some cases because the firm will pick up the remainder, regardless of the subsidies it qualifies for based on its average wage. Table 2-13 reflects our calculations of how the differences in employee and employer shares affect total contribution levels. We estimate that employers would contribute

Table 2-13. Estimated Premium Revenues for Adults Ages Eighteen to Sixty-Four[a]

Units as indicated

Revenue source	Income, by percent of FPL				
	<100	100–199	200–399	400+	Totals
Average percentage contribution from					
Employer	12.0	32.5	34.5	52.5	. . .
Individual	6.3	12.5	34.5	47.5	. . .
Government general revenue	81.8	55.0	31.0	0.0	. . .
Total contribution (billions of dollars) from					
Employer	8.3	28.6	52.2	87.8	176.8
Individual	4.3	11.0	52.2	79.4	146.9
Government general revenue	56.4	48.4	46.9	0.0	151.7
Total revenues (billions of dollars)	68.9	88.0	151.2	167.2	475.4

Source: Authors' calculations.

a. Numbers may not sum to totals due to rounding.

$176.8 billion, individuals $146.9 billion, and the federal government $151.7 billion.

Under Medicare Part E, the premium for a family earning $40,000 a year, after government and employer contributions, would amount to approximately 11 percent of its pretax income for health insurance for two adults with children. We apply our premium calculation in table 2-13 to estimate total revenues for the program but note that precise calculation would take into account the fact that firms are expected to cross-subsidize their lowest-wage workers. In addition, premium revenues for children under age eighteen will be equivalent to $26.7 billion, for total premium revenues of $502.1 billion. The federal government will pay $151.7 billion of this amount (table 2-13).

7. COST OFFSETS AND COMPENSATING FACTORS. We have not included a potentially significant source of savings that comes from the reduction in the rate of individuals being uninsured. An IOM study (2003b) estimates that the economic value of a lack of insurance coverage ranges from $1,645 to $3,280 per uninsured person per year—between $65 billion and $130 billion aggregated for the United States.[7] The IOM study also estimates the cost of increased financial risk to families without

7. Wilhelmine Miller, Elizabeth R. Vigdor, and Willard G. Manning, "Covering the Uninsured: What Is It Worth?" *Health Affairs,* web exclusive, March 31, 2004 (content. healthaffairs.org/cgi/reprint/hlthaff.w4.157v1).

insurance, calculating that this increased risk poses an aggregate economic cost of $1.6 to $3.2 billion for uninsured Americans (IOM 2003b). A more detailed study conducted in the state of Maryland found that expenditures by and for the uninsured in that state in 2003 totaled $1.47 billion dollars—equivalent to $2,371 per full-year uninsured person in the state (Waters and others 2007). Additionally, providers would see an increase in income as services previously provided on an uncompensated basis to the uninsured become reimbursable. The Lewin Group estimates that universal coverage would result in an increase in provider income of approximately $16.3 billion (Sheils and Haught 2003, appendix A).

What Is Not Included in the Cost Estimates

For the sake of clarity, these simulations employ several simplifications. First, medical inflation is not included. All cost estimates use 2006 dollars. Second, we do not account for pent-up demand—the expansion of insurance that leads to initial levels of utilization that are higher than normal because previously uninsured individuals use services that they wanted or needed earlier but could not afford. Third, as explained earlier, any potential federal subsidies to compensate for the effects of risk selection are not included.

Possible Concerns about Medicare Part E

The Medicare Part E proposal creates several analytical and political issues, including
—concerns over mandates that everyone must have health insurance coverage,
    —the impact of tax increases on labor market participation,
    —the potential crowd-out of private health insurance,
    —the effect of Medicare Part E on the existing Medicare program,
    —Medicare Part E's potential adverse impact on providers,
    —the ability of Medicare cost sharing to control spending,
    —coverage of undocumented immigrants,
    —concerns about Medicaid, and
    —alternative options such as the Federal Employees Health Benefit program, state initiatives, other Medicare expansion proposals, and proposals similar to Medicare Part E.
    In this section, we attempt to address these concerns.

Are Mandates Necessary?

Some have argued that mandates interfere with the marketplace and can have adverse employment effects. There is public concern over whether the benefits of universal coverage outweigh the costs of mandates, particularly for small employers.[8] Critics of the Medicare Part E proposal will assert that any mandate—employer or individual—will interfere with the marketplace and could lower employment, especially for low-wage workers. They might also argue that low-income individuals have more pressing needs than health insurance coverage, so low-wage workers cannot afford to pay anything for health insurance coverage.

We argue that mandates are necessary if everyone is going to obtain health insurance coverage and if the federal government is not going to provide the coverage directly. Previous attempts to provide financial inducements to employers or individuals to purchase health insurance have estimated that a considerable percentage of the uninsured would remain uninsured (Glied 2001).[9] One study showed that nine out of ten individuals who tried to get coverage through the individual market never bought a plan because coverage was unaffordable or because they were turned down (Collins and others 2006). According to estimates, providing a $7,500 tax deduction for individuals and a $15,000 tax deduction for families as proposed by President Bush may induce only a small proportion of the uninsured to obtain health insurance coverage (Collins, Davis, and Kriss 2007).

The Medicare Part E proposal attempts to minimize the impact of the mandates on low-income individuals. The amount an individual must pay is directly related to his or her income. While everyone with an income (as calculated by how much each person pays in Medicare taxes) will pay something, the percentage of the total premium is minimal for individuals with very low incomes. Only when the person's income reaches 400 percent of the FPL will that individual pay the full premium.

Medicare Part E also attempts to minimize the impact of the mandate on small businesses. They will receive considerable federal subsidies to help

8. Becky Bright, "Poll Shows Support for Measures on Employer Health-Insurance." *Wall Street Journal Online,* April 25, 2007 (online.wsj.com/article/SB117733987603679051. html?mod=dist_smartbrief).

9. See also Karen Davis, "The 2007 State of the Union Address: The President's Health Insurance Proposal Is Not a Solution," February 2007 (www.commonwealthfund.org/aboutus/aboutus_show.htm?doc_id=448217).

allay the cost of mandated health care, especially since they tend to hire a relatively high proportion of low-income workers. Part E also places workers in small businesses in a much larger insurance pool, reducing the risk selection problems that often lead private insurers to charge small businesses premiums that are not affordable.

Impact of the Proposal on Labor Market Participation

This proposal has the potential to affect the labor market in three ways. First, taxes will need to be increased to fund the annual subsidy. Second, for a family of four below 400 percent of the FPL, the phaseout of the premium subsidies is equivalent to raising the marginal tax rate by 12.5 percentage points. Finally, the employer mandate could affect employment if employers are not able to pass the cost of the mandate on to employees in the form of lower wages.[10] A caveat to the wage decreases and job loss due to insurance mandates is the potential benefit of providing health insurance to improve the health of employees. Better health translates to increased employee earnings, which could offset any wage loss due to the mandate.[11] Although this is a less researched area, evidence suggests that improving the health of employees increases productivity, reduces employee turnover, and decreases absenteeism for the firm (IOM 2003b).

Will Medicare Part E Crowd Out Private Health Insurance?

Private insurers are currently not marketing to the uninsured and would not choose to market to them in the absence of public dollars. Since the first Blue Cross plans were founded in 1929, the private sector has not found a viable way to insure the millions of Americans who do not have health insurance coverage.

Under Medicare Part E, private insurers could benefit and collect on previously uncompensated care costs that are currently absorbed through donated time, forgone profits, and philanthropy—an estimated $7.5 to $9.8 billion annually (Dobson, DaVanzo, and Sen 2006; Walker 2005;

---

10. Other common responses to mandates, such as shifting work to temporary or part-time workers, would be precluded because our proposal requires all workers to be covered regardless of work status. See Anna D. Sinaiko, "Employers' Responses to a Play-or-Pay Mandate: An Analysis of California's Health Insurance Act of 2003," *Health Affairs,* web exclusive, October 13, 2004 (content.healthaffairs.org/cgi/reprint/hlthaff.w4.469v1.pdf).

11. Jack Hadley, and John Holahan, "How Much Medical Care Do the Uninsured Use, and Who Pays for It?" *Health Affairs,* web exclusive, February 12, 2003 (content. healthaffairs.org/cgi/reprint/hlthaff.w3.66v1.pdf).

Direct Research 2003).[12] By recovering these costs, private insurers could lower their prices and attract additional subscribers.

A criticism of the Medicare Part E proposal is the crowd-out of private insurers if many individuals and firms choose to obtain Medicare Part E coverage. This will be a concern primarily of insurers that write policies to individuals and small firms. Unlike some other proposals that provide a new role for the private insurers, the Medicare Part E proposal does not automatically guarantee private insurers any additional roles. Several proposals have private insurers playing a major role, including the Massachusetts and California health care reform plans, America's Health Insurance Plans, the Federation of American Hospitals, and the Health Coverage Coalition for the Uninsured.[13]

Under Medicare Part E, the challenge for the private sector will be to develop innovative products in order to compete with Medicare for lower prices and better quality. If the private sector is able to create a better product than Medicare Part E, then it will be able to maintain its market share. If, as alleged, the Medicare fee-for-service benefit plan and payment system is outmoded, then it should be easy for the private sector to compete effectively with Medicare Part E.

The major arguments against guaranteeing a new role for private insurers are that they have higher administrative costs, have not demonstrated any greater efficiency in controlling spending increases, and are more likely to engage in risk selection. For these reasons, public funds should not be used to subsidize private insurers.

However, our proposal maintains three important roles for private insurers—Medigap, Part C, and Part D. The first is supplemental coverage. Currently, there are ten Medigap plans that are available to all Medicare

12. See also Jack Hadley and John Holahan, "How Much Medical Care Do the Uninsured Use, and Who Pays for It?" *Health Affairs,* web exclusive, February 12, 2003 (content. healthaffairs.org/cgi/reprint/hlthaff.w3.66v1.pdf).

13. See America's Health Insurance Plans (2004); Emanuel and Fuchs (2005); Gruber (2001); Holahan, Nichols, and Blumberg (2001); Kaiser Commission on Medicaid and the Uninsured (2006a); Kendall, Lemieux, and Levine (2002); Miller (2001); Singer, Garber, and Enthoven (2001). See also Federation of American Hospitals, "Health Coverage Passport: A Proposal to Cover All Americans," February 2007 (www.fah.org/passport/ HCP%20PPT%20Designed%202-16-07.pdf); Health Coverage Coalition for the Uninsured, "Expanding Health Care Coverage in the United States: A Historic Agreement," January 18, 2007 (www.familiesusa.org/issues/uninsured/hccu/hccu-agreement.pdf); Arnold Schwarzenegger, "Governor's Health Care Proposal," press release, January 8, 2007 (gov.ca.gov/pdf/press/Governors_HC_Proposal.pdf).

beneficiaries. These Medigap plans would also be available to the Part E beneficiaries, and it is likely that some Part E beneficiaries would choose to purchase them.

The second way that private health plans could participate is through the Part C program. If Part E were enacted, it would more than double the size of the Medicare program. This would allow more opportunities for health plans to participate in Medicare. The uninsured could be more likely than current Medicare beneficiaries to participate in Part C. The current Medicare beneficiaries are older, have more chronic conditions, have established relationships with doctors and other health providers, and may be more risk averse. The Medicare Part E beneficiaries will be younger, healthier, lack established relationships with most providers, and may find that the managed care options are a better match to their needs. As a result, a higher percentage of the currently uninsured could choose Part C. At present, most individuals in small firms have a limited choice of health plans; under Part E, employees would have more options and could choose to enroll in Part C.[14]

Medicare beneficiaries in Part E could also enroll in prescription drug plans under Medicare Part D. Under our proposal, almost 65 million new beneficiaries would purchase drug coverage under Part D, and the private sector would be able to compete for new business.

Our proposal does not require the private sector to provide as generous a benefit package as Medicare, so a potential concern is that some health plans would have to enrich their benefit packages.[15] Hopefully, health plans will be able to find ways to offer less expensive plans than Medicare Part E with equally good or better benefit packages.

In this proposal, the minimum benefit package that private insurers would have to offer in order to qualify is not very restrictive. High-deductible health plans, for example, would qualify. Firms that have employees that find this type of health insurance coverage acceptable would meet the requirement, and private insurers could continue to offer this option.

Many other proposals for universal health care have endorsed expanding programs that involve more generous benefit packages, such as Medic-

14. Kaiser Family Foundation, "Trends and Indicators in the Changing Health Care Marketplace" (www.kff.org/insurance/7031/index.cfm).

15. Joseph P. Newhouse, and Robert D. Reischauer, "The Institute of Medicine Committee's Clarion Call for Universal Coverage," *Health Affairs*, web exclusive, March 31, 2004 (content.healthaffairs.org/cgi/reprint/hlthaff.w4.179v1.pdf).

aid. However, we do not see an argument for why the uninsured should get better benefits than Medicare beneficiaries or many privately insured individuals.

Will Medicare Part E Adversely Affect the Existing Medicare Program?

We agree that the Medicare program needs modernization. The Medicare Modernization Act of 2003 (House of Representatives 2003) was an important first step. It began the much needed transformation of the Medicare program into one that is oriented to the needs of people with chronic conditions (Anderson 2005; Anderson and Chu 2007). We anticipate that additional changes will be forthcoming. Some of these changes are outlined in other chapters in this volume.[16]

A possible concern is that Part E would have an adverse impact on the Medicare program. On the contrary, Part E should strengthen the Medicare program. Medicare Part E is self-sustaining and is not permitted to run a deficit net of the income subsidies. Firms with large shares of unhealthy and low-wage workers, or individuals who are unhealthy or earn low wages, may be early adopters of Part E. Subsidies are built in for low-wage employees, and general revenues will be used for subsidization of firms with a large low-income population. Premiums may start high, but as more firms and individuals find Part E to be an affordable option compared to the private sector, premium growth will slow with the healthier and wealthier mix of beneficiaries in Part E.

In addition, Medicare Part E could actually strengthen the existing Medicare program by giving the program additional market power with providers. Data collected by the Medicare Payment Advisory Commission (2007) suggest that private insurers are paying substantially higher rates for physician services than does the Medicare program (figure 2-2). At the present time, the Medicare program cannot lower its payments too far below the rates paid by private insurers without jeopardizing access to care for Medicare beneficiaries. A larger share of the marketplace would allow the Medicare program greater ability to constrain the rates that it pays to providers.

Will Medicare Part E Have an Adverse Impact on Providers?

Providers continually complain about the low rates paid by the Medicare program. As shown in figure 2-2, Medicare rates are lower than the private

---

16. See Furman, chapter 7, and Lambrew, chapter 8.

Figure 2-2. Ratio of Private Insurer Physician Fees to Medicare Payment Rates, 1993–2005[a]

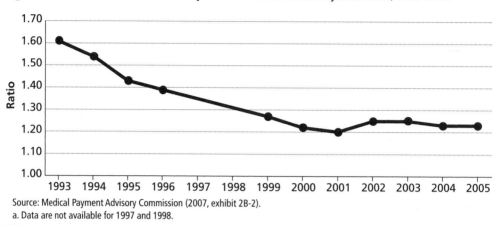

Source: Medical Payment Advisory Commission (2007, exhibit 2B-2).
a. Data are not available for 1997 and 1998.

sector. As a result, most providers would prefer options that involve the private sector.

Three arguments may persuade providers otherwise. The strongest argument is that providers, including hospitals, currently receive only a small portion of what they bill uninsured patients (Dobson, DaVanzo, and Sen 2006). Under this plan, providers would receive Medicare payment rates for individuals that previously paid very little. This will substantially improve the bottom line for many providers.

Second, Medicare rates are designed to allow the efficient health care provider a small profit (Direct Research 2003). Third, some providers also argue that the Medicare program forces them to incur greater administrative expenses than they incur with the private sector. However, the providers are already incurring these administrative expenses if they participate in the Medicare program. Once the providers have established the administrative apparatus to respond to Medicare rules and regulations, the marginal cost of treating additional Medicare beneficiaries will be relatively low.

Can the Medicare Program Control Spending?

The problems encountered by the Medicare program are well known. Spending is increasing at levels that cannot be sustained without significant changes in benefits, dramatic reductions in payments to providers, or tax increases (Fuchs and Emanuel 2005). Others have suggested that Medicare is not a reasonable option for covering the uninsured because of long-standing problems with the Medicare program.

However, private insurers have been even less successful at controlling health care spending than the Medicare program over the past thirty-five years. As noted earlier, evidence indicates that the private sector pays more than Medicare for identical services in the United States (Direct Research 2003). Indeed, the U.S. private market also pays higher prices for drugs and other services than the public sector pays in other countries.[17] Furthermore, under Medicare Part E, the actuaries would be required to set rates that ensure that the Medicare Part E program is self-sustaining over each year.

Another concern is that the Medicare program relies heavily on regulation and stifles the marketplace. One problem with this argument is that international experience suggests that the marketplace is not effective at controlling health spending. Switzerland and the United States have two of the most expensive health care systems in the world; both countries rely heavily on private markets (Anderson and others 2006; Herzlinger and Parsa-Parsi 2004; Reinhardt 2004). If the health insurance market were able to obtain less expensive alternatives, then health care expenditures would be lower in these two countries. At the same time, while payments to providers in the United States are higher, there is no evidence that clinical outcomes are better or that satisfaction is higher in countries where the health care system is more market oriented (Anderson and others 2003; Hussey and others 2004; Reinhardt, Hussey, and Anderson 2004; World Health Organization 2000).[18] International comparisons seem to suggest that the health care market is ineffective at controlling costs and providing quality care. And to the point here, the U.S. market has also failed to develop any solutions to cover the uninsured.

Finally, the Medicare Part E option provides important opportunities for the private sector. Part E will more than double the number of individuals participating in the Medicare program, thus doubling the number of individuals that might choose one of the Part C or Part D alternatives.

17. It has been shown that the United States pays much higher prices than other comparable countries do for most goods and services used in health care. See Anderson and others (2003). See also Gerard F. Anderson and others, "Doughnut Holes and Price Controls," *Health Affairs,* web exclusive, July 21, 2004 (www.healthaffairs.org/RWJ/Anderson.pdf).

18. See also Cathy Schoen and others, "Primary Care and Health System Performance: Adults' Experiences in Five Countries," *Health Affairs,* web exclusive October 28, 2004 (content.healthaffairs.org/cgi/reprint/hlthaff.w4.487v1).

An effective private health plan should be able to compete with the Medicare fee-for-service program and not incur the marketing expense.

What about Undocumented Immigrants?

According to the last census, there were an estimated 9.6 to 9.8 million undocumented immigrants in the United States, or approximately 25 percent of the uninsured (Camarota 2005). However, another estimate is that as few as 6 to 7 percent of nonelderly uninsured are undocumented immigrants, given that 21 percent of the nonelderly uninsured are noncitizens and 30 percent of 36 million immigrants in the United States are undocumented.[19]

Undocumented immigrants will not be automatically covered under this proposal. However, Medicare Part E would be available to anyone who pays the Medicare tax. This would provide health insurance coverage for many undocumented immigrants because they are currently paying into the Medicare program.

Certain classes of nonresident foreign nationals on temporary visas in the United States who are currently exempt from Social Security and Medicare taxes would continue to be exempt.[20] They would be able to use the U.S. system, but payment would be arranged as under current law. However, as current law also specifies, spouses and dependents of nonresident aliens are subject to Social Security and Medicare taxes if they are employed; thus these individuals would be eligible to enroll in Medicare Part E.

The current safety net would continue to operate. Those undocumented immigrants that contribute to Medicare would get health insurance coverage, and the remaining undocumented immigrants would not be any worse off. If migrant workers are granted guest worker status as a result of immigration reform, and if they pay Medicare taxes, then they could fall under any new individual or employer mandates.

Why Not Medicaid?

The United States has a number of publicly funded health care financing and delivery systems. For purposes of this discussion, they will be divided

---

19. Estimate provided by Kaiser Family Foundation based on data found at www.pewhispanic.org.

20. Nonresident aliens include nonimmigrant students, scholars, teachers, researchers, trainees, physicians, au pairs, summer camp workers, and other nonimmigrants who are in the United States temporarily under F-1, J-1, M-1, Q-1, or Q-2 visas.

into two main categories: financing systems and delivery systems. We will quickly dismiss the delivery systems as a viable alternative because they do not actually provide health insurance coverage. Individuals covered under these systems would still need to be enrolled in Medicare Part E or be covered by the private sector.

Service delivery programs such as those provided by the Veterans Health Administration or the Health Services and Resources Administration (for example, community health centers) are important programs that provide care to both insured and uninsured populations. They will need to be maintained to supply care for individuals with special health care needs and for undocumented immigrants. Under this proposal, the workload from undocumented immigrants will likely diminish because the uninsured will obtain health insurance coverage and thus better access to medical care. However, since Medicare Part E would only be available to individuals paying taxes for the Medicare program, there will remain a need for free or low-cost providers for undocumented immigrants and nonresident aliens.

Turning now to the financing options, there are three publicly financed models available: Medicare, Medicaid, and state-only options. Each option has been proposed as a mechanism to cover the uninsured. In ensuing discussion, the advantages and disadvantages of each option are compared, and the reasons why we prefer the Medicare option are explained.

Expanding the Medicaid program is often suggested as a method for covering the uninsured (America's Health Insurance Plans 2004; Feder and others 2001; Pauly 2001).[21] Some of the reasons are historical—local provision of care to the poor is traditional in English law, and states were chosen as the embodiment of local provision in Title XIX (Grants to States for Medical Assistance Programs) of the Social Security Act. Another reason is that the Medicaid program is oriented to the provision of care for the poor.

However, there are several compelling reasons not to choose Medicaid as the primary vehicle for covering the uninsured. First, the Medicaid program has a very generous benefit package—much more generous than Medicare and most private sector insurers. While a generous benefit package would seem desirable for the recipients, and while there are clear gaps

---

21. See also Federation of American Hospitals, "Health Coverage Passport: A Proposal to Cover All Americans," February 2007 (www.fah.org/passport/HCP%20PPT%20Designed%202-16-07.pdf); Health Coverage Coalition for the Uninsured, "Expanding Health Care Coverage in the United States: A Historic Agreement," January 18, 2007 (www.familiesusa.org/issues/uninsured/hccu/hccu-agreement.pdf).

in the Medicare benefit package, choosing the Medicaid benefit package would be considerably more expensive and raise the total cost of covering the uninsured. The added expense of Medicaid would partly be due to the inclusion of long-term care coverage and limited cost sharing. As discussed earlier, we find this unappealing in part because expanding Medicaid would likely require raising provider payments. Furthermore,, it would be politically difficult to give the uninsured a better benefits package than that of Medicare recipients and most privately insured people. It would increase pressure on the Medicare program and on the private sector to expand their benefits packages, thereby increasing total health care spending. These changes would be necessary to make an expanded Medicaid sustainable, but they would also increase the cost considerably.

A second problem is that each state has a different Medicaid benefit package. This would mean that the benefits that the uninsured would receive would vary from state to state. If the state was financially supporting the coverage of the uninsured, then using the Medicaid program as the vehicle for covering the uninsured is understandable. However, under Medicare Part E, the state does not contribute its own funds.

A third problem with using the Medicaid program as the primary vehicle for providing insurance to the currently uninsured is the low rates that many Medicaid programs pay to providers. These low rates are extremely unpopular with doctors, hospitals, and other providers. For this reason, a universal Medicaid option would be less popular among health care providers.

A fourth problem is that Medicaid is a federal-state partnership with both the states and the federal government contributing to the program. Under most proposals to cover the uninsured (including Medicare Part E), the state government is not actually contributing to the cost of covering the uninsured. Funding comes from the federal government; states are not expected to contribute their own resources. When the federal government is providing all the funds, it is unclear why the states necessarily need to be involved.

A fifth problem with a Medicaid expansion that retains a federal-state partnership is that states have different percentages of uninsured. Table 2-14 shows, as of 2005, the eight states with the highest percentage of uninsured (where two states are tied for second place and four states tied for fifth place) and the five states with the lowest percentage of uninsured.[22]

22. Kaiser Family Foundation, "Health Insurance Coverage of the Total Population, States (2004–05), U.S. (2005)" (statehealthfacts.org).

Table 2-14. Distribution of Uninsured, 2005

Percent

Geographic unit	Uninsured rate
United States	15
Top eight states	
Texas	24
Florida	20
New Mexico	20
Oklahoma	19
Arizona	18
California	18
Georgia	18
Nevada	18
Bottom five states	
Pennsylvania	10
Wisconsin	10
Hawaii	9
Iowa	9
Minnesota	8

Source: Kaiser Family Foundation, "Trends and Indicators in the Changing Health Care Marketplace," April 11, 2005 (www.kff.org/insurance/7031/index.cfm).

If the differences in the percentage of uninsured were solely due to differences in state policies and spending, it might be acceptable for states to bear different cost burdens under a federal mandate for universal coverage. Nevertheless, many factors contribute to differences in the percentage of uninsured, not the least of which is the difference in the characteristics of residents among states. As such, there is little justification for why some states should pay a higher burden than other states to cover the uninsured.

Finally, some have proposed moving all low-income, nonelderly, and nondisabled individuals to Medicare, but our goal is to make the least number of changes while achieving the greatest amount of coverage. Moving this population to Medicare would require a payroll opt-out that is hard to implement. Tracking who is insured by what firm in a dual-worker family would also be difficult. It would require compliance reporting above and beyond what Medicare already does, which would add to the cost of the proposal. Also, moving current Medicaid beneficiaries to Medicare would make some individuals worse off.

Why Not the Federal Employees Health Benefit Program?

Another option is the Federal Employees Health Benefit (FEHB) plan. This plan is used to cover government workers, including members of

Congress. The FEHB plan is often used as a model for covering the uninsured (Collins, Davis, and Kriss 2007). There are, however, several problems with using FEHB to cover the uninsured.

First, there is an unclear benefits package in FEHB. About half of beneficiaries are enrolled in a Blue Cross–Blue Shield plan under FEHB; the rest are in a variety of other managed care plans. Each plan participating in FEHB has a different benefit structure and uses a different payment system to pay providers.

Our second concern is similar to the earlier argument about adopting Medicaid: we do not see a convincing reason for providing the uninsured with a more generous benefit package than Medicare provides. The third issue is that using Blue Cross–Blue Shield as the blueprint for a benefits package and for payment structure gives one private insurer additional market power compared to other private insurers. Fourth, the payment rates paid under FEHB are typically higher than Medicare rates, leading to an increase in the cost of covering the uninsured. Finally, there is a private sector choice for individuals who want something other than fee-for-service Medicare—Medicare Part C.

Why Not State Initiatives?

Another alternative is to enroll the uninsured in state health insurance programs. These could be the plans that are offered to state government workers or other programs established by the states.

Hawaii has the longest operating program to cover the uninsured; recently a number of states have either passed or are considering legislation to cover their uninsured. The primary advantage of this approach is that states are often a laboratory for federal government health care initiatives and programs.

However, there are many problems with relying on states to cover the uninsured. First, Employee Retirement Income Security Act (ERISA) rules generally prevent states from involving large employers, which often have more resources than small employers. Since in most states more than half of the employed population works in firms covered by ERISA, this limits the state's ability to get the largest and often the most affluent employers to contribute to covering the uninsured. A second and related problem is that many firms are multistate. This means that they can move their office, plants, and facilities to whichever state does not mandate health insurance coverage. Perhaps the most compelling argument against state-specific solutions, however, is the uneven burden across the United

States in the number of uninsured. Table 2-14 has already shown the variation in the percentage of uninsured across the states. As a result, some states have greater burdens than other states. Nevertheless, the problem of the uninsured is primarily national and not local.

Why Not Other Medicare Expansion Proposals?

There are a variety of proposals and federal legislation that have proposed covering everyone under Medicare (House of Representatives 2006a, 2006b, 2007). The Medicare for All Act (House of Representatives 2006b), for instance, would have insured everyone in the United States through the Medicare program. This would have entailed a fundamental change in how health care is delivered in the United States. Even some of the supporters of this option agreed that it is more of a concept than a realistic alternative (Hacker 2006).

One problem with the Medicare for All Act was that the tax increases necessary to support the U.S. health care system primarily though public financing would have been politically and economically unacceptable. The total health care spending in the United States in 2010 is projected to be $2.8 trillion. The Congressional Budget Office (2007) projects total federal revenues in 2010 to be $2.9 trillion. If health expenditures were totally supported by the federal government, nearly all the federal tax revenues in 2010 would have to be allocated to health care—clearly an unacceptable option. In subsequent years, health spending would exceed all government revenues.

Perhaps more important is that the current system works reasonably well for the wealthy and the healthy. These individuals would sharply oppose any attempt to replace their current private health insurance with Medicare coverage because many of them would pay higher taxes but receive a less generous benefit package.

Similar Proposals to Medicare Part E

In 1991 Karen Davis recommended the expansion of Medicare to cover the uninsured (Davis 1991). The benefit package of Davis's plan would have a reduced deductible and limits on cost sharing compared to the current Medicare program. Employers would contribute at least 6 percent of workers' wages to the expanded Medicare program or to a private health insurance plan with similar benefits. Employees and all other uninsured individuals would contribute 2 percent of their family income to health care coverage, which is unfavorable for high-income individuals and families. Under the Davis proposal, states would have the option to buy into Medicare for all of their Medicaid beneficiaries. Low-income individuals would be subsidized through an earned income tax credit. Financing Davis's plan would require restructuring the Medicare trust funds and changing the current Medicare Part B premium settings. Davis's plan would be funded through premium contributions and state Medicaid funds if states decide to buy into Medicare.

Medicare Plus, developed by researcher Jacob Hacker, is a variation of the Davis proposal, with a few key differences (Hacker 2001). The benefits include a single deductible and wraparound services for those that have moved from Medicaid and SCHIP. Medicare Plus limits the role of private health insurers by requiring the prescription drug benefit to be provided directly by the Medicare Plus program. Employers are required to provide benefits as generous as Medicare Plus or else pay an approximate 5 percent payroll tax to participate in Medicare Plus. However, employees instead may take the employer contribution minus a penalty and purchase a private health plan with similar coverage. The movement of low-income individuals combined with the option of employees to opt out of Medicare Plus sets up the program for serious adverse risk selection.

In 2006 Congress debated an option similar to Medicare Part E. The AmeriCare Health Care Act (House of Representatives 2006a) proposed expanding the current Medicare program while maintaining a role for private health insurers. It covered individuals not covered by employer-sponsored health insurance, as well as all low-income adults and children not receiving long-term care under Medicaid—effectively dismantling the Medicaid and SCHIP programs. AmeriCare was to be funded by premiums, state funds previously earmarked for Medicaid, and general revenues. The AmeriCare benefit package was more generous than the Medicare program, with lower deductibles and out-of-pocket caps, and cost sharing was not required for children, individuals, and families below 200 percent of the FPL. AmeriCare provided a sliding-scale subsidy only up to 300 percent of the FPL. Employers were required to cover all of their employees with a benefit package equivalent to AmeriCare or else pay 80 percent of the premium cost for AmeriCare coverage for their employees.

Most of these proposed plans, while similar to Medicare Part E in building on a well-established Medicare program, make significant changes to the current Medicare program as well as to two other public programs, Medicaid and SCHIP. The Medicare Part E program does not make these changes and focuses simply on covering the uninsured.

Conclusion

Medicare Part E(veryone) achieves universal coverage by offering the current Medicare benefits to everyone. Part E is simple to understand and easy to implement since the plan builds on existing infrastructure. Employers can buy into the plan or keep their current private insurance. Families under 400 percent of the FPL receive subsidies—an aspect of the plan that also helps keep costs down for small businesses. Although there will still be room for improvement in the health care system, Medicare Part E provides a fiscally sensible way to achieve affordable, universal, and continuous health insurance coverage.

References

America's Health Insurance Plans. 2004. *Board of Directors Statement: A Commitment to Improve Health Care Quality, Access, and Affordability.* Washington.

Anderson, Gerard F. 2005. "Medicare and Chronic Conditions." *New England Journal of Medicine* 353, no. 3: 305–09.

Anderson, Gerard F., and Edward Chu. 2007. "Expanding Priorities: Confronting Chronic Disease in Countries with Low Income." *New England Journal of Medicine* 356, no. 3: 209–11.

Anderson, Gerard F., and others. 2003. "It's the Prices, Stupid: Why the United States Is So Different from Other Countries." *Health Affairs* 23, no. 3: 89–105.

———. 2006. "Health Care Spending and Use of Information Technology in OECD Countries." *Health Affairs* 25, no. 3: 819–31.

Biles, Brian, and others. 2006. "The Cost of Privatization: Extra Payments to Medicare Advantage Plans—Updated and Revised." Issue paper. New York: Commonwealth Fund (November).

Blendon, Robert J., and others. 2006. "Americans' View of Health Care Costs, Access, and Quality." *Milbank Quarterly* 84, no. 4: 623–57.

Camarota, Stephen A. 2005. "Immigrants at Mid-Decade: A Snapshot of America's Foreign-Born Population in 2005." Backgrounder. Washington: Center for Immigration Studies (December).

Claxton, Gary, and others. 2006. *Employer Health Benefits: 2006 Annual Survey.* Chicago: Kaiser Family Foundation and Health Research and Educational Trust.

Collins, Sara R., Karen Davis, and Jennifer L. Kriss. 2007. "An Analysis of Leading Congressional Health Care Bills, 2005–2007: Part I, Insurance Coverage." Report. New York: Commonwealth Fund (March).

Collins, Sara R., and others. 2006. "Squeezed: Why Rising Exposure to Health Care Costs Threatens the Health and Financial Well-Being of American Families." Publication 953. New York: Commonwealth Fund (September).

Congressional Budget Office. 2007. *The Budget and Economic Outlook: Fiscal Years 2008 to 2017.*

Davis, Karen. 1991. "Expanding Medicare and Employer Plans to Achieve Universal Health Insurance." *Journal of the American Medical Association* 265, no. 19: 2525–28.

Direct Research. 2003. *Medicare Physician Payment Rates Compared to Rates Paid by the Average Private Insurer, 1999–2001.* Final report prepared for the Medicare Payment Advisory Commission.

Dobson, Allen, Joan DaVanzo, and Namrata Sen. 2006. "The Cost-Shift Payment 'Hydraulic': Foundation, History, and Implications." *Health Affairs* 25, no. 1: 22–23.

Dubay, Lisa, John Holahan, and Allison Cook. 2007. "The Uninsured and the Affordability of Health Insurance Coverage." *Health Affairs* 26, no. 1: w22–w30.

Emanuel, Ezekiel J., and Victor R. Fuchs. 2005. "Health Care Vouchers: A Proposal for Universal Coverage." *New England Journal of Medicine* 352, no. 12: 1255–60.

Feder, Judith, and others. 2001. "Public Coverage Expansion with Employer Tax Credit." In *Covering America: Real Remedies for the Uninsured,* edited by Eliot K. Wicks. Washington: Economic and Social Research Institute.

Fuchs, Victor R., and Ezekiel J. Emanuel. 2005. "Health Care Reform: Why? What? When?" *Health Affairs* 24, no. 6: 1399–414.

Glied, Sherry A. 2001. "Challenges and Options for Increasing the Number of Americans with Health Insurance." *Inquiry* 38, no. 2: 90–105.

Glied, Sherry A., Dahlia K. Remler, and Joshua G. Zivin. 2002. "Inside the Sausage Factory: Improving Estimates of the Effects of Health Insurance Expansion Proposals." *Milbank Quarterly* 80, no. 4: 603–35.

Gruber, Jonathan. 2001. "A Private/Public Partnership for National Health Insurance." In *Covering America: Real Remedies for the Uninsured,* edited by Eliot K. Wicks, pp. 59–71. Washington: Economic and Social Research Institute.

Hacker, Jacob. S. 2001. "Medicare Plus: Increasing Health Coverage by Expanding Medicare." In *Covering America: Real Remedies for the Uninsured,* edited by Eliot K. Wicks, pp. 75–100. Washington: Economic and Social Research Institute.

———. 2006. "Universal Insurance: Enhancing Economic Security to Promote Opportunity." Policy Brief 2006–07. Brookings, Hamilton Project (September).

Hadley, Jack. 2003. "Sicker and Poorer: The Consequences of Being Uninsured: A Review of the Research on the Relationship between Health Insurance, Medical Care Use, Health, Work, and Income." *Medical Care Research and Review* 60, no. 3: 3S–75S.

Hadley, Jack, and John Holahan. 2003–04. "Is Health Care Spending Higher under Medicaid or Private Insurance?" *Inquiry* 40, no. 4: 323–42.

Herzlinger, Regina E., and Ramin Parsa-Parsi. 2004. "Consumer-Driven Health Care: Lessons from Switzerland." *Journal of the American Medical Association* 292, no. 10: 1213–20.

Hoffman, Earl D., Jr., Barbara S. Klees, and Catherine A. Curtis. 2004. "Brief Summaries of Medicare and Medicaid: Title XVIII and Title XIX of the Social Security Act." Baltimore: Centers for Medicare and Medicaid Services (November).

Holahan, John F., Allison Cook, and Lisa Dubay. 2007. "Characteristics of the Uninsured: Who Is Eligible for Public Coverage and Who Needs Help Affording Coverage?" Issue Paper 7613. Washington: Kaiser Commission on Medicaid and the Uninsured.

Holahan, John F., Len M. Nichols, and Linda J. Blumberg. 2001. "Expanding Health Insurance Coverage: A New Federal/State Approach." In *Covering America: Real Remedies for the Uninsured,* edited by Eliot K. Wicks, pp. 103–18. Washington: Economic and Social Research Institute.

Hussey, Peter S., and others. 2004. "How Does the Quality of Care Compare in Five Countries?" *Health Affairs* 23, no. 3: 89–99.

Institute of Medicine (IOM). 2001. *Coverage Matters: Insurance and Health Care.* Consequences of Uninsurance series. Washington: National Academy of Sciences.

———. 2002a. *Care without Coverage: Too Little, Too Late.* Consequences of Uninsurance series.

———. 2002b. *Health Insurance Is a Family Matter.* Consequences of Uninsurance series.

———. 2003a. *A Shared Destiny: Community Effects of Uninsurance.* Consequences of Uninsurance series.

———. 2003b. *Hidden Costs, Value Lost: Uninsurance In America.* Consequences of Uninsurance series.

———. 2004. *Insuring America's Health: Principles and Recommendations.* Consequences of Uninsurance series.

Kaiser Commission on Medicaid and the Uninsured. 2006a. "Massachusetts Health Care Reform Plan. Key Facts." Publication 7494. Washington.

———. 2006b. *The Uninsured: A Primer. Key Facts about Americans without Health Insurance.* Report 7451. Washington.

Kendall, David B., Jeff Lemieux, and S. Robert Levine. 2002. "Federal Tax Credits with State Coverage Responsibility." In *Covering America: Real Remedies for the Uninsured,* vol. 2, edited by Eliot K. Wicks, pp.. Washington: Economic and Social Research Institute.

Medicare Payment Advisory Commission. 2007. "Section 2B: Physician Services." In *Report to the Congress: Medicare Payment Policy* (March).

Miller, Edward, Jessica Banthin, and John Moeller. 2004. "Covering the Uninsured: Estimates of the Impact on Total Health Expenditures for 2002." Working Paper 04407. Rockville, Md.: Agency for Healthcare Research and Quality.

Miller, Robert H., and Harold S. Luft. 1994. "Managed Care Plan Performance since 1980: A Literature Analysis." *Journal of the American Medical Association* 271, no. 19: 1512–19.

———. 1997. "Does Managed Care Lead to Better or Worse Quality of Care?" *Health Affairs* 16, no. 5: 7–25.

———. 2002. "HMO Plan Performance Update: An Analysis of the Literature, 1997–2001." *Health Affairs* 21, no. 4: 63–86.

Miller, Tom 2002. "Improving Access to Health Care without Comprehensive Health Insurance Coverage: Incentives, Competition, Choice and Priorities." In *Covering America: Real Remedies for the Uninsured,* vol. 2, edited by Eliot K. Wicks, pp. 39–59. Washington: Economic and Social Research Institute.

Pauly, Mark V. 2001. "An Adaptive Credit Plan for Covering the Uninsured." In *Covering America: Real Remedies for the Uninsured,* edited by Eliot K. Wicks, pp. 137–52. Washington: Economic and Social Research Institute.

Reinhardt, Uwe E. 2004. "Regulated Competition without Managed Care." *Journal of the American Medical Association* 292, no. 10: 1227–31.

Reinhardt, Uwe E., Peter S. Hussey, and Gerard F. Anderson. 2004. "U.S. Health Care Spending in an International Context." *Health Affairs* 23, no. 3: 10–25.

Sheils, John, and Randy Haught. 2003. *Cost and Coverage Analysis of Ten Proposals to Expand Health Insurance Coverage.* Washington: Economic and Social Research Institute.

Singer, Sara J., Alan M. Garber, and Alain C. Enthoven. 2001. "Near-Universal Coverage through Health Plan Competition: An Insurance Exchange Approach." In *Covering America: Real Remedies for the Uninsured,* edited by Eliot K. Wicks, pp. 155–71. Washington: Economic and Social Research Institute.

U.S. House of Representatives. 2003. *Medicare Modernization Act of 2003.* H.R. 1. 108 Cong. 1 sess.

———. 2006a. *AmeriCare Health Care Act of 2006.* H.R. 5886. 109 Cong. 2 sess.

———. 2006b. *Medicare for All Act.* H.R. 4683. 109 Cong. 2 sess.

———. 2007. *United States National Health Insurance Act.* H.R. 676. 110 Cong. 1 sess.

Walker, David M. 2005. "Nonprofit, For-Profit, and Government Hospitals: Uncompensated Care and Other Community Benefits." Testimony before Committee on Ways and Means, House of Representatives. GAO-05-743T. U.S. Government Accountability Office.

Waters, Hugh, and others. 2007. "The Costs of Non-Insurance in Maryland." *Journal of Health Care for the Poor and Underserved* 18, no. 1: 139–51.

World Health Organization. 2000. *The World Health Report 2000.* Health Systems: Improving Performance.

Evolving beyond Traditional Employer-Sponsored Health Insurance

3

STUART M. BUTLER

Access to adequate and dependable health insurance is one of the keys to economic security. When health coverage is uncertain or unafford-able, workers and their families face broad economic consequences and suffer personal anxiety. For most working-age families in the United States, health coverage is directly connected to the workplace. So the availability or absence of employment-based health insurance and the structure and cost of benefits when insurance is available affect basic employment decisions. Coverage, or the lack thereof, influences the choice between full-time or part-time employment and the decision whether to work in one company or another. Workers with medical problems may find themselves locked into a job, unable to switch to a better job or start their own business because they dare not give up their current benefits. And older, sicker employees may feel forced to put off retirement or have difficulty finding reemployment if they lose a job. The present structure for delivering health coverage thus influences countless employment decisions, weakening the economic security of households and the efficiency of the labor market.

In addition to these effects on families with insurance, the current employment-based system fails to deliver the goal of adequate and secure

The author thanks Stan Dorn and Edmund Haislmaier for insightful comments on earlier drafts and Greg D'Angelo for research assistance.

Figure 3-1. Percent of Nonelderly Americans with Employment-Based Coverage

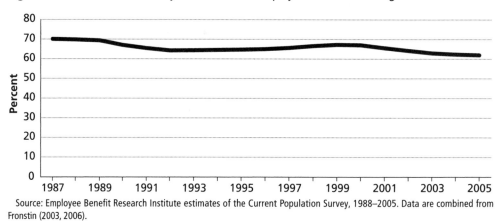

Source: Employee Benefit Research Institute estimates of the Current Population Survey, 1988–2005. Data are combined from Fronstin (2003, 2006).

health coverage for all of the working population. The Census Bureau, using revised data for 2005, reports that 44.8 million people, or 15.3 percent of the population, lacked health insurance in that year. The unrevised data, which provide more specific breakdowns, show that 17.7 percent of all full-time and 23.5 percent of all part-time employees were uninsured (DeNavas-Walt, Proctor, and Hill 2006, p. 22). In fact, although most nonelderly Americans continue to receive health insurance through their place of work, the percentage has been falling over the last two decades while the proportion who are uninsured has been rising. According to an Employee Benefit Research Institute analysis of Census Bureau data (figure 3-1), the share of nonelderly Americans with employer-sponsored coverage has been declining steadily in recent decades, from 70.1 percent in 1987 to just 62.0 percent in 2005. Over that same period the proportion of nonelderly Americans without coverage climbed from 13.7 percent to 17.9 percent (Fronstin 2003, 2006).

It is time to recognize the structural weaknesses inherent in the traditional vision of employment-based health insurance and to take steps to allow the employment-based system to evolve into a sounder model that matches more closely the needs of today's workforce. The model proposed in this chapter is based on state-chartered exchanges within which commercial insurers and other entities would offer health insurance to workers and their families. In this model, the employer typically would no longer be a *sponsor* or manager of benefits but instead a *facilitator* of coverage, handling premium payments and arranging tax relief for its insured employees.

The availability of coverage, the choice of plan, and the availability of tax subsidies no longer would depend on the employer's decisions about insurance. Instead a separate system of sponsorship and coverage infrastructure would become available in the form of the insurance exchange. For those satisfied with the traditional system of employer-sponsored insurance, that form of coverage would remain: the current role of the employer as both sponsor and facilitator of insurance could continue where it works reasonably well. In either case, employers would continue to play a central role in making health insurance available.

Three key steps are needed to achieve this transformation in the employment-based system in a gradual way that avoids disrupting its successful elements. First, states should establish insurance exchanges. Exchanges would make available an array of coverage options to working families. Use of a single, statewide insurance exchange would allow families to retain their chosen plan as they move from workplace to workplace, enjoying the same tax benefits as families in traditional employer-sponsored plans.

Second, employers should become facilitators, but not necessarily sponsors, of insurance coverage. Sponsorship of insurance is a very different function from the management of payments. These should generally be separated. So while many large employers would continue to sponsor coverage, most employers would hand that task over to the insurance exchange and focus on providing administrative support for their employees' insurance choices.

Third, the federal government should reform the tax treatment of health insurance. While the first two steps would significantly improve the choice and portability of insurance obtained through the workplace, combining these steps with reform of the tax treatment of health benefits would make coverage even more affordable and available to low-paid working families. Specifically, the federal government should gradually phase in greater tax relief for insurance coverage (whether sponsored by an employer or obtained through an exchange) to lower-income families and less to upper-income households than under current law.

These three steps would trigger a natural evolution of the current, employment-based system, enabling it to adjust to the requirements of today's workforce and the widely differing capabilities of employers to organize health insurance. And by rationalizing the system of tax subsidies for health coverage while creating new options for families to obtain permanent, dependable, and portable coverage of their choice, these steps would speed progress toward the goal of universal coverage.

Box 3-1. Why We Have Employer-Sponsored Health Insurance Today

America's employer-sponsored insurance system is unique among major countries: even Germany's work-based coverage is centered on industries rather than firms. Only in America are coverage and access to health care so dependent upon one's place of work. This system did not come about as the result of a consensus vision or explicit legislation. Although employers here, as in other countries, have always been concerned about maintaining a healthy workforce, an employer-sponsored system would not have begun, much less persisted, without three related developments:

—wage controls imposed during World War II, which provided an incentive for employers to offer and employees to accept uncontrolled fringe benefits, including health coverage, because benefits were not subject to controls;

—a series of tax rulings, later codified in the landmark 1954 federal tax law, that exempted such benefits from taxation, providing a major tax advantage for employer-sponsored coverage; and

—a 1948 ruling by the National Labor Relations Board that health benefits were a legitimate subject of collective bargaining, further spurring the growth of employment-based coverage, especially in unionized firms.

For a detailed discussion of these developments, see Glied and Borzi (2004).

Why the Time for Traditional Employer-Sponsored Insurance Has Passed

America's employer-sponsored insurance arrangements took root as the result of a series of regulatory accidents rather than as a conscious strategy to design an optimal health system (see box 3-1). Nevertheless, the system has proved popular over the years, and advocates of this peculiarly American arrangement claim a number of advantages on its behalf.

One is that the workplace is said to be a particularly good location for pooling insurance risks for group coverage. People typically join a firm's workforce for reasons other than the availability of health insurance. Employment-based pools thus have a degree of randomness in the distribution of risk within the group. This makes them in principle less prone to adverse selection, in which less healthy individuals gravitate toward more generous insurance plans, raising the group premium and thus inducing healthier participants to leave, raising premiums further and triggering a "death spiral" of ever-rising premiums. Another claim is that employers provide administrative economies of scale so that the cost of managing workplace-based health insurance is lower than that of providing group insurance in other ways and much lower than for individual insurance. A third claim is that employers are effective agents for employees and their families in the health care marketplace. Americans routinely pick a trusted agent, such as a financial adviser or a realtor, to help them make complex decisions or to act as their intermediary in obtaining a service. The purchase of health insurance is likewise a difficult decision, and employers are said to have particular advantages in organizing health coverage for families. Many firms have entire personnel and benefits departments that routinely negotiate benefits with service providers and can tailor coverage to employees' needs, either directly or within collective bargaining.

On the face of it, employment-sponsored insurance does seem to have these attractive characteristics. But it also has some severe and inherent shortcomings, particularly in the case of smaller employers and in certain sectors of the economy. In addition, the tax treatment of health insurance and certain other policies governing health care has some distorting features that lead to costly inequities and obstruct the development of better coverage arrangements. The rest of this section details some of the flaws in the employment-based insurance system. Although these flaws do not imply that the system should be dismantled, they should prompt a reexamination, followed by action, to permit this part of the health care system to evolve in a new direction.

Increasing Worker Mobility

The increasing mobility and changing nature of the workforce have significantly weakened the traditional argument for employer-sponsored insurance as the foundation for coverage for working families. That argument implicitly assumes that these families have a strong and continuous link with a single place of employment. But this is becoming less and less the case in the United States. As the U.S. Department of Labor (2006, especially chapters 3 and 6) notes, not only has there been a steady shift in recent decades of workers from the goods-producing sector to the services sector, where labor turnover is higher, but American workers today generally change employers more frequently. Today as much as a quarter of the workforce changes jobs every year. In addition, whereas in 1983 almost two-thirds of men in their fifties had spent ten or more years with the same employer, by 2004 that fraction had fallen to just over half. Work arrangements are also changing. During the last decade, for instance, the number of workers with alternative employment arrangements (such as independent contractors) increased by over 20 percent, to about 11 percent of the workforce, and today about 17 percent of the workforce is part-time.

This increasing mobility in the workforce and the correspondingly looser employer-employee relationship mean that employer-sponsored insurance is less able to provide working families with continuous, portable coverage. Americans do not have to requalify for their mortgage or their life insurance when changing jobs, but they do face gaps or changes in health coverage. Even if they obtain comparable coverage with another employer, that is not true portability: they may have to give up a preferred physician or switch from one drug to another that may not deal as well with their condition. And although the federal government, in enacting the Consolidated Omnibus Budget Reconciliation Act (COBRA) in the 1980s and the Health Insurance Portability and Accountability Act (HIPAA) in the 1990s, has sought to cushion such disruptions in employer-sponsored coverage, these laws do not ensure meaningful portability. HIPAA does not ensure continuity of physician or other benefits for some-one who leaves an employer, nor does it ensure that any new coverage will be affordable. Neither HIPAA nor COBRA coverage normally qualifies for tax relief, and so workers who leave a job can find continuous coverage prohibitively expensive.[1]

Declining Employer Sponsorship of Health Insurance

Employers meanwhile are becoming far less dependable sponsors of insur-ance for their employees, and many do not sponsor it at all. Worse still, in some parts of the economy, employer-sponsored coverage is especially sparse. In particular:

—Coverage is poor or nonexistent in small firms. An inherent problem with making the employer the basis of an insurance risk pool is that the smaller the employer, the less the pool represents a good, random mix of the general population with respect to health risk. This actuarial problem, which compounds the administrative hassles and low economies of scale facing small employers considering health coverage, results in low cover-age rates in smaller firms. While, for instance, 78.9 percent of workers and dependents in private sector firms of 1,000 or more had employer-sponsored coverage in 2005, the figure was only 48.4 percent in firms with fewer than 10 employees and only 50 percent among self-employed households. More than 35 percent of workers in firms with fewer than 10 employees were uninsured in 2005, compared with only 13.4 percent in firms employing 1,000 or more (Fronstin 2006, p. 11).

---

1. For a discussion of portability problems see Goodman (2006).

—Most very small firms offer no coverage at all. A large proportion of workers in certain types of firms are not even offered insurance. According to the Employee Benefits Research Institute, data from the Census Bureau's Survey of Income and Program Participation for 2002 indicate that 54.1 percent of uninsured employees were not offered insurance by their employer (Fronstin 2005, p. 15). Firm size is the dominant factor. The annual survey of employers conducted by the Kaiser Family Foundation and the Health Research and Education Trust (2006, section 2, p. 4) found that in 2005 only 48 percent of firms with 3 to 9 employees and 73 percent of firms with 10 to 24 employees offered coverage at all, compared with 98 percent of firms employing 200 or more. Another Kaiser study found that almost half the decline in adults with employer-sponsored insurance during 2001–05 was due to employers (typically small firms) dropping coverage (Clemens-Cope, Garrett, and Hoffman 2006, p. 6).

This gradual erosion of employer-sponsored insurance reveals two very different worlds. In the largest firms, employers generally continue to be stable sources of coverage for workers and their dependents (although some families, largely because of inequities in the tax subsidy system, do not take advantage of it). But in the small business sector, and especially the lower-wage services sector, uncertainty and huge gaps in the coverage available for employees prevail.

Tax Inequities and Perverse Incentives

The tax treatment of employer-sponsored insurance creates huge inequities and perverse incentives. A major culprit is the excludability of employer-provided health benefits. Employers receive a tax deduction for contributing to insurance coverage for their employees, as they do for most other forms of employee compensation. But the health insurance part of an employee's total compensation is also excludable without limit from the employee's taxable income: workers pay no income or payroll tax on this employment-based health insurance. This is a huge tax break. Thomas Selden and Bradley Gray (2006) estimated the total revenue loss associated with this tax treatment in the personal tax code at $208.6 billion, of which the federal income tax and payroll tax components were $111.9 billion and $73.3 billion, respectively (state income tax subsidies accounted for the remaining $23.4 billion).

But this tax benefit has two inequitable features. First, only those employees whose employer selects and pays for their insurance receive it. The millions of working families whose employer does not sponsor their health coverage are ineligible for this large subsidy, even if they purchase their own insurance, and even if the employer makes a financial contribution to the employee but does not sponsor coverage directly.[2] These workers must pay for coverage with after-tax dollars.

Second, the tax benefit is highly skewed toward employees in higher tax brackets, who typically also have more generous coverage. Selden and Gray (2006) put the average tax subsidy per covered employee at $2,778. But in firms where more than half the employees are low wage (under $10.43 an hour), the average subsidy per enrolled worker was just $2,268, while for firms where more than half were classified as high wage (more than $23.07 an hour), the subsidy was $3,283, almost 45 percent higher. Furthermore, the remaining, unsubsidized portion of an employee's health insurance is a far larger share of income for lower-income employees, leading many to decline the offer of coverage and thus forfeit the subsidy. The actual subsidy per worker for *eligible* (but not necessarily enrolled) workers in low-wage firms averaged just $673. Analyzing the subsidy by family income, John Sheils and Randall Haught estimated that in 2004 families with incomes of $100,000 or more received an average health tax subsidy of $2,780, compared with an average of $1,448 for families with incomes between $40,000 and $50,000, and just $102 for families earning less than $10,000.[3] Some 26.7 percent of all federal tax expenditure for health insurance went to families earning $100,000 or more, while 28.4 percent went to families with incomes below $50,000—similar proportions, but the latter group is four times as numerous (57.5 percent of families versus 14 percent).

This inequitable subsidy aggravates the general erosion of health benefits among lower-income families, especially within the small business sector. With the price of health insurance rising faster than wages, employers considering insurance as part of the compensation package now face a bill for family coverage amounting to one-third or even a half of the total compensation they might provide to a low-skilled worker. The economic reality is that firms that do provide health coverage must offset the cost by offering stagnating or even declining cash wages to these workers. If these workers benefited from a generous tax subsidy for their health insurance, that could offset the impact of depressed wages. But without such a sub-

2. The tax code does offer a limited deduction for self-employed individuals and certain deductions for out-of-pocket employee spending.

3. John Sheils and Randall Haught, "The Cost of Tax-Exempt Health Benefits in 2004," *Health Affairs*, web exclusive, February 15, 2004 (content.healthaffairs.org/cgi/reprint/hlthaff.w4.106v1.pdf).

sidy, employer-paid coverage is becoming increasingly unsustainable for lower-income families. Meanwhile economists point out that because the after-tax price of employer-sponsored group insurance to an individual does not closely reflect that individual's usage of services, there is an incentive for covered employees to press for more extensive benefits and to use insured services but little or no incentive for them to seek cost-effectiveness in their insured medical care. The result is faster-rising health costs, making health care less affordable for both insured and uninsured families.[4]

Flaws in the Employer-as-Agent Model

Some employers, particularly very large employers with a stable workforce and a sophisticated health benefits department, are effective agents for their employees in the health care marketplace. But the wide spectrum of employer arrangements and the gaps in the system suggest it is time to rethink that role. Among small firms and in the services sector, which, as noted, have relatively high employee turnover, employers may desire to provide good treatment benefits so as to reduce absenteeism but have little incentive to invest in the long-term health of their employees or their dependents if the employee is likely to leave the firm in a few years. That helps explain why, for example, among firms that do offer insurance, only 49 percent of smaller firms (those with fewer than 200 workers) include dental benefits, while 80 percent of larger firms do (Kaiser Family Foundation 2006, exhibit 2.6).

A corollary is the phenomenon of "job lock." Consider an employee with a high-cost medical condition that is covered by the employer's insurance; such an employee may feel unable to leave the employer for a better job because the same coverage might be unavailable with a new employer. Federal law does give such employees the right to acquire individual coverage, but there are no restrictions on the cost they may face. Furthermore, the employer is ultimately the agent of its owners, not its employees. In the case of publicly owned corporations, the rising cost of health care and the financial condition of the firm itself inevitably force management to weigh the health care interests of its employees and their families against the business interests of the firm and its stockholders.

---

4. For a discussion of the relationship between low levels of cost sharing and rising health care spending, see Furman (2007). See also Antos (2006) and Steuerle (House of Representatives 2004).

The Health Exchange Plan: Initiating the Evolution of the Employment-Based System

The structural weaknesses of the employer-sponsored insurance system just outlined—increasing mobility of the workforce, rising pressure of health care costs on employers, inequities and perverse incentives in the tax treatment of health coverage, and the inability of many employers to serve as effective agents for their employees—are likely to get worse over time. As they do, they not only will increase the burdens and anxieties of those who remain insured but also will exacerbate the problem of uninsurance—the tens of millions who do without. Recognizing these inherent problems, the reform proposed in this chapter seeks to restructure the employer-based insurance system. This reform, called the Health Exchange Plan, would

—Create large, stable insurance groups for all workers so as to spread insurance risks more widely. Insurance pools for workers in small or medium-sized firms need to be much larger and more stable over time. Insurance plans could then be made available to working families through these pools to reduce risk and minimize adverse selection.

—Organize coverage that is continuous and portable between jobs. For coverage to become truly portable and continuous, it must be controlled and effectively owned by the worker. That requires two things. First, the favorable tax benefits associated with coverage must no longer be conditioned on the employer selecting, controlling, and owning an employee's coverage. And second, coverage should be available through a trusted sponsor or agent other than a person's employer so that a family can keep its chosen insurance plan as its worker members move from employer to employer and when they are between jobs.

—Transform most employers, especially small and medium-size firms, from sponsors of health insurance into facilitators of health insurance. It is time for a fundamental change in the role of the employer in health care, so as to separate the choice of insurance plan and organizing functions from the role of facilitating payments and paperwork. All employers should facilitate their employees' coverage decisions by arranging premium payments, adjusting tax withholdings, and perhaps contributing directly to an employee's chosen plan. But only in those cases where a firm and its employees prefer the employer to be the agent should employers continue to sponsor coverage.

—Make tax subsidies for health care fairer and more efficient. Reforming the more than $200 billion in federal and state tax breaks available annually could substantially increase the proportion of working families able to afford coverage. That will require targeting the tax benefit far more efficiently to those who really need it. It must also be made more equitable, so that similarly situated people receive similar tax support toward obtaining coverage, irrespective of whom they work for or where they get their coverage.

The Health Exchange Plan is predicated on the conviction that the health insurance system needs a bottom-up evolution, not a top-down revolution. The goals of the transformed system just described could, in principle, be reached through a comprehensive reform of the health insurance system for working families, for example, through sweeping changes in the tax treatment of health care and a national restructuring of the insurance market. But there are reasons why such a "revolution" approach would not be wise.

For one thing, as President Bill Clinton discovered in his efforts to transform the system in the mid-1990s, Americans are quite conservative about their health care. They may tell pollsters that they think the current system needs a complete overhaul, but those with coverage are simultaneously reluctant to see big changes in that coverage, other than to make it cheaper.[5] In the health insurance domain, it is important to introduce change gradually so that people with coverage can adapt.

It would also be unwise to change direction sharply because health care constitutes about one-sixth of the nation's economy, and any major change in the foundations of the employment-based part of the system would have large and complex effects that cannot be predicted with certainty. In addition, a sudden and complete transformation of the tax treatment of health insurance, even if beneficial, would lead to big changes in the tax liability of families and likely would trigger political concern and opposition. So, although it is important to have certain strategic goals as a compass, it makes sense both to proceed gradually and to allow a variety of approaches in different places to be tried and compared. Thus it also makes sense for the states rather than the federal government to take the lead in designing reform, to foster such experimentation and variety. That is how policymakers will best learn to address the complexities of insurance design and health care arrangements.

5. See, for example, Robert J. Blendon, John M. Benson, and Catherine M. DesRoches, "Americans' Views of the Uninsured: An Era for Hybrid Proposals," *Health Affairs,* web exclusive, August 27, 2003 (content.healthaffairs.org/cgi/reprint/hlthaff.w3.405v1.pdf); Robert J. Blendon and others, "Understanding the American Public's Health Priorities: A 2006 Perspective," *Health Affairs,* web exclusive, October 17, 2006 (content.health affairs.org/cgi/content/abstract/hlthaff.25.w508v1).

The first steps of the transformation should focus primarily on those who are served least well by the current system, namely, working families in the small business sector. Creating a framework that meets the needs of those Americans is most urgent and would provide a working model for others to consider embracing. To be sure, transformation should not be limited to small firms at this early stage. But if it appears successful and attractive for small firms, that would increase the probability that workers and employers in other firms would likewise accept reform, encouraging the rest of the employment-based system to follow.

What would a transformed employment-based system look like ten or twenty years from now? It is impossible to say with certainty because the exact complexion of employment-related coverage would change over time to reflect household preferences and the manner in which employers adapt to the changes. The proposed reform envisions an employer-as-facilitator arrangement (typically for small and medium-size firms) operating in parallel with the traditional employer-as-sponsor model. But the relative importance of these two types of arrangements in the transformed system is hard to predict. It might turn out that the employer-as-facilitator model is a major improvement for most workers but that the traditional employer-sponsored system continues to be more attractive for others, such as those who work for very large firms, where the goals of the proposed transformation are already largely in place for long-term employees (see box 3-2).

Whatever the pattern turns out to be, the proposed reforms would enable employment-related coverage to adapt in ways that it cannot today. And however the employer-based system changes over time, taking the proposed steps would enable the system to become a pathway to universal coverage rather than an obstacle to that goal.

Three sets of government actions are required to enable the current employer-based system to evolve into a system that incorporates the goals discussed above. First, states should establish "insurance exchanges" to enable families to select their coverage from a wide range of choices and to retain their chosen plan from job to job. Within this structure, religious, civic, and other organizations should be allowed to function both as plan sponsors and as agents. Second, states and the federal government should introduce rule changes and incentives to encourage employers, especially small employers, to become facilitators of health insurance for their employees. Third, the federal government should gradually reform the tax treatment of health care spending. Specifically, it should cap the tax exclusion for employer-sponsored health insurance and gradually transform the exclusion into a refundable tax credit for health coverage.

Box 3-2. Summary of Proposed Policy Changes

Create Insurance Exchanges

States would charter the exchanges under state law, much as they now charter such special-purpose nongovernmental entities as state universities. The state would determine such things as the infrastructure for handling premiums and the regulations governing entry requirements, and the operation of plans in the exchange, as well as establishing pooling and risk adjustment mechanisms. The state would decide whether or not to make the exchange the sole place through which commercial health insurance could be sold to individuals and employer groups. The federal government, through regulation or statute, would clarify that employer contributions to an exchange have the same tax-free compensation status for employees as contributions to a traditional employer-sponsored plan.

Establish a System of Employers as Facilitators

States would establish procedures whereby premiums collected through payroll deductions would be transmitted to the insurance exchange.

The federal government would require firms using an exchange to adjust employee tax with-holding to reflect available tax relief, and to establish payroll deduction arrangements compatible with the state insurance exchange's premium aggregator system.

Reform the Tax Treatment of Health Insurance

The federal government would cap the present tax exclusion for employer-sponsored insurance and create a refundable, advanceable, and assignable tax credit for lower-income families.

Establishing Insurance Exchanges

Under the proposed Health Exchange Plan, states would charter insurance exchanges under state law, much as they now charter special-purpose non-governmental entities such as state universities. These exchanges would in effect be market clearinghouses within which insurance providers would compete to offer workers portable health plans within a framework of standardized administrative procedures and uniform insurance rules (see figure 3-2). Each insurance exchange would thus function much like a stock exchange, in that the exchange does not itself sell the stock or the health plan but rather provides the venue and regulates the offerings and transactions.

Each state would determine on its own such features as the infrastructure for handling premiums, as well as the regulations and requirements for accepting insurance plans into the exchange. The state also would be responsible for determining pooling, reinsurance, and risk adjustment arrangements and the degree to which firms would, if at all, be required to

Figure 3-2. How the Health Exchange Plan Would Work

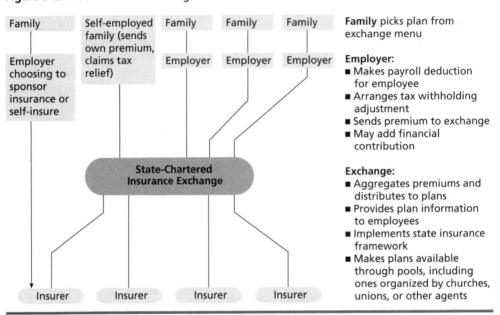

offer plans available through the exchange to their employees. Some employers would be exempt from such state requirements, notably those sponsoring insurance under federal Employee Retirement Income Security Act (ERISA) regulations, and could continue to sponsor insurance in the same way that they do today if they chose to do so.

Workers eligible for traditional employer-sponsored coverage would not be able to join plans offered through the exchange as individuals. They would have to obtain coverage through their employer and so could obtain an exchange plan only if their employer was using the exchange.

The federal government would encourage the use of such exchanges by clarifying that employees obtaining coverage from firms using the exchanges would enjoy the same tax breaks as employees with traditional employer-sponsored insurance.

Employer-sponsored insurance was intended to provide stable group health insurance. But as discussed earlier, for millions of Americans it fails to do so efficiently or, in many cases, at all. To deal with these short-comings and ensure group coverage that spreads risk and keeps premiums stable, insurance arrangements meeting certain key criteria are needed. One criterion is that the groups created be large enough for the group rate to be stable and predictable, not constantly fluctuating because sometimes a small number of its members incur unusually high medical expenses. Another criterion is that groups be reasonably stable in terms of risk composition over time. If people with medical risks well above the group median migrate into the group, or if healthier people migrate out, it can destabilize the group, leading to a spiraling of rates. Voluntary insurance associations are particularly vulnerable to adverse selection, as sicker people join in order to save money, and healthier people leave because the now-rising group rate makes individual coverage more attractive. A third criterion is true portability: workers should typically be able to retain the coverage that is right for their family even if they change jobs.

States can best ensure these characteristics by establishing insurance exchanges that offer stable, portable coverage through large groups for those workers and their families who currently lack such coverage.

An exchange is important to achieving a transformed system because it does two things. First, it provides what have been described as the "market organizer" and "payment aggregator" functions needed so that working families without adequate coverage today can obtain coverage that mimics the best features of traditional large-employer coverage (see Haislmaier and Owcharenko 2006). And second, designing the exchange to dovetail with federal employee benefit law makes possible a seamless facilitator role for employers. Various forms of exchanges have been proposed, such as those suggested by Alain Enthoven.[6]

Although states do not need federal legislation to create exchanges, explicit clarifications of federal rules would encourage states to establish them. Under today's federal law, for instance, employees pay no income or payroll tax on compensation in the form of an employer contribution to an employer-sponsored health plan. A U.S. Treasury ruling or a declaratory federal law stating that the same tax exemption would apply to any contributions toward coverage made through a qualified state health insurance exchange would remove any lingering uncertainty for states. Such a ruling or law would relieve the employer and the exchange of having to go through the legal artifice of the employer "sponsoring" a separate "plan" and the exchange contracting to "administer" the plan. There should be additional federal regulatory or statutory clarifications in other areas, such as the application of nondiscrimination rules to employer contributions for

---

6. See Alain C. Enthoven, "Employer-Based Insurance Is Failing: Now What?" *Health Affairs,* web exclusive, May 28, 2003 (content.healthaffairs.org/cgi/reprint/hlthaff.w3. 237v1?). See also Singer, Garber, and Enthoven (2001).

coverage in an exchange where plans are sold on an age-rated basis (that is, with different premiums for participants of different ages).

Insurance exchanges would not be costly to implement because in reality they would merely take over and centralize the existing sponsorship functions of the typical large firm, and the administrative costs could be factored into the price of insurance offered through the exchange.

EXISTING MODELS. Models currently exist of what insurance exchanges would look like and how they would function. The state of Massachusetts made an insurance exchange, which it dubbed the "Commonwealth Connector," a core part of its new health insurance system, and other states are developing similar legislation (Haislmaier and Owcharenko 2006). The Federal Employee Health Benefits Program (FEHBP), an older example of an exchange at the national level, covers about 8 million federal employees as well as retirees. Although technically a traditional employer-sponsored program (the employer being the federal government), the FEHBP in practice works like a giant exchange with complete plan portability across the various federal agencies and congressional offices.

The Office of Personnel Management (OPM) administers the FEHBP. Once OPM has approved a wide range of national and local plans, it is the employee or retiree, not his or her immediate employer (a member of Congress, say, or a federal judge, a federal agency, or even the U.S. Postal Service), who chooses the plan. The government makes a significant tax-free contribution to each plan, and the OPM handles the administrative details. Plans must meet certain basic conditions and must provide the OPM with standardized information on their benefits and terms. OPM then distributes enrollment information to beneficiaries and manages the premium collections and payments to plans. Although many of the FEHBP plans are available only in certain areas, and some are restricted to certain categories of employees, most federal workers have access to the same wide range of plans, whether they work in a small congressional office or a huge agency, and they can retain the same plan if they switch federal jobs or retire.

As Edmund Haislmaier and Nina Owcharenko (2006) explain in their discussion of the health exchanges developing in Massachusetts and other states, the basic insurance exchange structure has several important features that make it more practical than the traditional employer-sponsored alternatives. First, it makes coverage more available and portable. Once an employer makes the exchange its "employee welfare benefit plan" for purposes of federal law, the firm's workers and their dependents have access to the plans available through the exchange, which enjoy the same tax and

Figure 3-3. How Portability Is Achieved under the Health Exchange Plan[a]

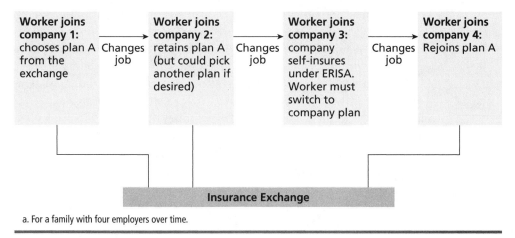

| **Worker joins company 1:** chooses plan A from the exchange | Changes job → | **Worker joins company 2:** retains plan A (but could pick another plan if desired) | Changes job → | **Worker joins company 3:** company self-insures under ERISA. Worker must switch to company plan | Changes job → | **Worker joins company 4:** Rejoins plan A |

Insurance Exchange

a. For a family with four employers over time.

other benefits as employer-sponsored coverage. These benefit plans are made available by but not run by the employer. So, if an employee switches jobs, he or she can retain the previously chosen plan without restriction (see figure 3-3). The firm does not have to negotiate with plans or create its own self-insured plan, as under traditional employer-sponsored insurance. Firms can also prorate coverage contributions for part-time employees, with the expectation that the worker will be able to get full coverage directly through the exchange and fund the balance of the premium out of other family earnings, most likely from another job held by the employee or his or her spouse. Self-employed individuals can also join directly simply by virtue of being a resident of the state.

Second, it acts as a premium aggregator. In the FEHBP, the premiums for each worker's chosen plan are deducted from the worker's paychecks and combined with the government subsidy for federal employees, and the aggregate amounts are transferred by OPM to the insurance providers. This sharply reduces the paperwork and other complexities for federal employees and for individual federal offices and agencies. In addition, OPM provides plan information to employees and organizes an annual "open season," during which employees can switch plans. The exchange system proposed here would include a similar "premium aggregator" and informational role. For employers participating in its exchange, Massachusetts is creating a uniform payroll withholding system that operates much like federal and state tax withholding and like OPM's system for the

FEHBP. In this way administrative costs can be reduced, and the exchange's responsibility as a clearinghouse reduces the payment risk that insurers build into their premiums.

Third, it provides a framework for insurance rules and pooling. Plans offered through an exchange, like plans offered through the FEHBP, have to comply with a set of state insurance rules (federal in the case of the FEHBP) intended to make coverage affordable, portable, and consistent. To maximize the effectiveness of an exchange in helping manage risk for plans and for families, states would have to set uniform minimum benefit and rating standards as well as procedures for handling high-risk individuals. States also would enact laws governing carrier solvency, actuarial sufficiency (Are the premiums to be charged for the plan likely to cover the expected benefit payments?), and market conduct (such as the insurance provider's business practices for offering coverage and handling claims).

Finally, it increases the availability of plans offered by trusted agents. The exchange provides a framework in which plans can be offered not only by commercial insurers but also by not-for-profit organizations acting as sponsoring agents. Just as union-sponsored plans are available under the FEHBP, so plans sponsored by unions, religious groups, and other organizations could be offered through an exchange. Exchanges would foster such trusted-agent plans for several reasons. For one thing, with plans contracted through exchanges deemed equivalent for tax purposes to employer-sponsored plans, the tax disadvantage faced by such plans when sold in the current individual market would disappear. For another, an exchange with a risk adjuster would minimize the adverse selection bias for or against a plan that appealed to a particular social group, and so organizations with generally sicker or healthier groups would not destabilize the market. The same would be true of plans that tended to attract individuals with certain specific medical conditions based on data showing that they do a superior job of managing the costs and outcomes associated with that condition.

THE CRITICAL FEDERAL ROLE. The federal government has a critical role in facilitating state insurance exchanges by making it clear that employees obtaining coverage through the exchanges would enjoy the same tax breaks as employees with traditional employer-sponsored insurance. The federal government has already indicated that state exchanges meet the requirements of an employee welfare benefit plan, with the exchange deemed the plan administrator. And the Treasury has indicated that money collected by an employer and sent to an exchange carries the same tax benefits for an employee as money for an employer-sponsored plan. Thus the federal government appears to treat a plan obtained through an exchange much like one obtained through the FEHBP. But to remove any remaining uncertainty or ambiguity, either the Treasury should issue a clear ruling on the tax treatment of contributions to an exchange, or Congress should enact clarifying language.

THE CENTRAL ROLE OF EMPLOYERS. The Health Exchange Plan envisions employers as the access point to the insurance exchange. But the proposal is compatible with various ways of accomplishing this, from voluntary contracts with the exchange to a state mandate for certain classes of firms to take part.

Self-employed individuals could join the exchange directly, and in principle it would be reasonable to allow non-self-employed workers to join directly as well. There are good reasons, however, for a state to make employee access contingent on whether the employer contracts with the exchange to provide coverage.

One reason is that employers have become efficient facilitators of payments. If policymakers had decided to construct an exchange system before the advent of employer-sponsored insurance, they might well have chosen to allow all working families to join directly. But decades of employer involvement in benefits have created an infrastructure of payroll deduction procedures, tax withholding, and other roles for the employer that makes the place of employment a practical entry point for health insurance, even in the case of small firms.

In addition, the experience with payroll deductions for pensions and health coverage indicates that even if employees are not required to sign up, making it easy to do so at the workplace does increase the probability that the employee will take the offered benefits. So, in keeping with the vision of the employer as a facilitator, there is good reason on behalf of families to encourage employers, even small firms, to designate an exchange as their source of coverage and so make that coverage more accessible for their employees.

LIMITING ADVERSE SELECTION. Gaining employer acceptance of exchanges also requires steps to limit the threat of adverse selection. An employer who willingly provides insurance today will understandably worry that if individual employees have the ability and incentive to pick and choose between the firm's group coverage and another arrangement, adverse selection could undermine the employer's group plan. The fear of adverse selection is a reason why employers who offer coverage often resist tax credit proposals or other proposals they fear would induce healthier employees to pull out of their plan.

The need to limit such adverse selection underscores why the Health Exchange Plan envisions employers as the point of entry to the exchange system, with states determining the details. Firms currently regulated under ERISA would not be required to take part in state-initiated exchanges and could continue their current forms of coverage—but they could join if they wished. That is why the employer decides whether or not all its employees will have access to the exchange, and why employees with employer-sponsored insurance would be allowed to use the proposed tax credit only for that coverage, if it is available. Over time, however, one might expect more and more employers to opt for an exchange as their designated source of coverage as they and their employees come to see the advantages.

Employers as Facilitators, Not Sponsors

Under the Health Exchange Plan, employers choosing to use the exchange, or required to do so under state law, would have two key functions: handling their employees' tax relief, and organizing the collection and payment of premiums to the exchange. Accordingly, employers using an exchange would be required under federal law to do two things. First, they would have to adjust employee tax withholdings to provide employees with tax relief for payments made to the exchange. Second, they would have to arrange an automatic payroll deduction and payment system, much as many do today for flexible spending accounts or for savings plans such as 401(k) retirement plans and 529 college savings plans. This deduction system would have to be linked to the payment aggregator system administered by the exchange for premium payments.

For those typically larger firms that choose to continue to sponsor insurance under ERISA or within the bounds of state insurance law, there would be no change and no new requirements.

Creating an insurance exchange with the same tax benefits to employees and employers as traditional employer-sponsored insurance would allow employers to delegate most insurance selection and management—the health care human resource functions—to the exchange. They would retain only the basic bookkeeping functions that make the workplace a convenient and efficient location to sign up for health insurance or for savings plans.

This separation of employer sponsorship and facilitating functions would be good for employees since it would increase their choice of tax-advantaged plans by providing access to plans available through trusted agents in the exchange rather than only plans selected by the employer.

Families with plans obtained through a state insurance exchange would also gain the certainty and true portability of coverage that millions of working families lack today.

The separation would also be good for employers. While the typically larger firms that are comfortable with traditional plan sponsorship could continue to organize and manage employee coverage, other employers could avoid those headaches. Yet they would also have an important new way of providing health benefits via the workplace—benefits that would typically be more attractive than those available through the vast majority of firms today, with expanded choice and improved portability. By delegating the cumbersome sponsorship functions, these employers could then focus greater attention on their core business activities. In addition, with the exchange itself distributing the insurance risk associated with higher-risk families, employers opting for the exchanges would have few or no concerns about potential medical problems associated with new hires.

Separating the sponsorship and facilitation functions would actually make it more attractive for smaller firms to make coverage available to employees and even to contribute to it. With the exchange available as a source of coverage, small firms could offer access to a range of coverage that is normally unthinkable for them to offer today. And free of the administrative complexity and selection risk, many such firms likely would decide to contribute to comprehensive benefits (for example, through a defined financial contribution) rather than struggle to offer less adequate benefits themselves as they often do today.

It is important, however, to appreciate that a system based on employers as facilitators rather than as sponsors is not the same as moving in the direction of defined contributions: the facilitator role refers to a separate mode of coverage and is compatible with either a defined-contribution or a defined-benefit model. For firms and employees pursuing a defined-contribution arrangement, the exchange, together with the employer in its facilitator role, would enable workers to steer such contributions toward a plan that is portable and most in line with their needs. But combining an exchange with an enhanced facilitator role for employers also would enable those firms committed to defined benefits—especially smaller firms with limited insurance expertise—to offer portable coverage and greater choice. The reason is that, within this framework, an employer can still commit to financing the actuarial value of a specified benefit package while allowing the employee to select an exchange-sponsored plan with employer funds based on the cost of a defined benefit. In effect, the FEHBP works in this way since the government commits to a contribution based on the premium cost of specific benchmark plans, and so the contribution is indexed to specific benefits rather than to a defined cash contribution.

DELIVERING TAX RELIEF THROUGH WITHHOLDING. The facilitation role would be nothing new for firms. Employers of all sizes today are required by federal law to carry out such a role in the tax system. They must distribute IRS (and typically state) tax withholding forms to workers, deduct appropriate amounts from paychecks for payroll and income taxes, and remit the money to the government. When the employee claims tax deductions and credits, such as a mortgage deduction, a child credit, or the Earned Income Tax Credit, the employer must adjust the withholding accordingly. But although employers facilitate the operation of the tax system in America, they do not sponsor it. And even smaller firms neither face undue hardship in carrying out the withholding obligation nor serve as tax accountants or advisers for their employees.

Under the Health Exchange Plan, the only change would be that this requirement to adjust tax withholdings would also apply to contributions made to a health insurance plan within an exchange. Employers would have to adjust for whatever federal and state tax relief applied, including any new tax credits (see below). The burden on employers would be minimal. A recent major survey sponsored by the Commonwealth Fund found that 76 percent of large employers and 88 percent of small firms (those with 3 to 199 workers) expressed willingness to administer a tax withholding mechanism to deliver a tax credit (Whitmore and others 2006, exhibit 3, p. 1673).

COLLECTING AND REMITTING PREMIUMS THROUGH PAYROLL DEDUCTIONS. Employers of all sizes commonly act as facilitators for their employees who contribute to retirement and other savings plans, such as 401(k) and 529 plans. The employer arranges a payroll deduction, adjusts the tax withholding, and in many cases also makes a financial contribution. A critical feature of such employer-facilitated savings plans is that they are portable: the plan and its tax benefits follow the employee from one employer to the next, and the plan remains with the employee if he or she leaves the workforce.

Under the Health Exchange Plan, employers could and should facilitate portable, tax-preferred health insurance in a similar way. If a state established an insurance exchange and an employer made the exchange available to its employees—either voluntarily or as required by the state—federal law would require that employer to arrange a payroll deduction system for the employees and to make payments to the exchange on their behalf. In turn, the exchange would provide standardized and unbiased information on available health plans, in accordance with its obligations under federal law as the plan administrator. Workers would pick the plan they wished, and the employer would consolidate and remit regular payments to the exchange, making appropriate adjustments to each worker's paycheck after adding whatever financial contribution the employer had agreed to make. The exchange then would aggregate the premium payments and disburse them to the plans according to their enrollments.

Although a requirement to establish a payroll deduction system would be a new obligation for some firms, particularly very small ones, the burden has been sharply reduced in recent years thanks to improved computer technology and the ready availability of contract payroll management companies. Perhaps not surprisingly, then, the Commonwealth Fund survey also found strong employer willingness to set up payroll deduction arrangements to assist employee enrollment in non-employer-sponsored coverage. Some 73 percent of large firms and 88 percent of small firms expressed willingness to organize payroll deductions to pay the premiums for government-administered health programs (Whitmore and others 2006).

Reforming the Tax Treatment of Health Insurance

Under the Health Exchange Plan, Congress would enact a cap on the existing unlimited exclusion of employer-sponsored insurance from taxable income while also phasing in a refundable, advanceable, and assignable tax credit for lower-income families. Amounts above the cap would become taxable for employees above a certain income. The cap would be indexed each year to the consumer price index (CPI). Workers eligible for the credit could use it only for health insurance. They would have to use it for plans offered through a state insurance exchange if their employer made the exchange available to them. If instead their employer sponsored coverage, they would have to use it for that insurance.

The changes proposed so far would be important steps toward the goal of health care security for working American families through a rationalized employment-centered system. Delinking the sponsorship of coverage from the facilitation of coverage at the workplace would lead to significant improvements in the availability of coverage through a gradual evolution of the current system. Delinking the existing tax breaks for health coverage from direct employer sponsorship would also be a significant step toward a fairer and more efficient tax subsidy system. It would achieve greater "horizontal" tax equity: tax benefits would become more similar for comparable families in different employment situations.

But even with these improvements in horizontal equity, the "vertical" inequities would remain. The tax treatment of health care would still provide large subsidies to upper-income families with generous employer-sponsored insurance, and inadequate or no subsidies to lower-income families struggling to afford even modest insurance. Thus reforming the tax treatment of health insurance is the third key piece of the reform equation. Although structural tax reform is not necessary for the evolution of today's employment-based system into a postindustrial model, it would sharply increase the new model's ability to provide health security to lower-paid working Americans.

Economists and health analysts broadly agree on the general outlines of a desirable reform of the tax treatment of health insurance. On one side of the tax ledger, reformers would taper down, and some would eventually end, the personal income tax exclusion for employer-sponsored health insurance, at least for upper-income households. This would reduce the importance of health insurance as a tax-free fringe benefit or eliminate it altogether. But to make the tax subsidy for health coverage more equitable, reformers would simultaneously phase in a tax credit for health insurance, whether obtained from the employer or from other sources. In this way the tax subsidy would gradually be refocused onto those who most need help and would no longer be confined to employer-sponsored insurance.

Several large-scale versions of this restructuring have been put forward as legislative or policy proposals, including by this author (Butler 2001). Because of the impacts of the current tax breaks on tax revenue and household incomes, however, any large-scale and rapidly implemented reforms would involve significant transfers of tax benefits and significant disruption. Those major financial effects, in tandem with the general reluctance of Americans to countenance rapid change in their health care situation, make a radical redesign of the tax treatment of health care over a short period unwise. More gradual and limited steps are needed.

PLACE A CAP ON THE TAX EXCLUSION. Under the Health Exchange Plan, Congress would enact a gradually tightening cap on the value of the tax exclusion for employer-sponsored health insurance while simultaneously introducing a tax credit for low-income families. The value of sponsored benefits above the cap would be taxed as cash compensation for families above a certain income. Such a reform could be made revenue neutral over time. Or it could involve new net tax benefits. Or it could be designed to achieve a net reduction in the projected growth of the tax subsidy, which could help to dampen the escalation of health costs generally, yielding potential savings in public as well as private health care costs (see Antos and Rivlin 2007).

The cap would be set high enough to initially affect only a relatively small proportion of Americans, thereby limiting the political resistance. However, the cap would be indexed at a rate lower than the current antici- pated cost escalation of employer-sponsored coverage, such as the CPI, so that over time a steadily larger number of employees would be affected. The cap in the plan offered in 2007 by President Bush ($15,000 for family coverage and $7,500 for individuals) may be unduly high (the average fam- ily plan costs approximately $11,000) but is probably more politically achievable in the short term than a tighter limit.

Under the proposal, the value of plans offered to employees in excess of the cap would become taxable only for households above a certain thresh- old income, in the same way that a portion of Social Security benefits is taxable above a certain income. Families with more modest incomes could enjoy comprehensive coverage and still not be affected. The income thresh- old would not, however, be indexed. The combination of a CPI-indexed cap and a nonindexed income threshold means that, over time, an increas- ing proportion of plans and households would be subject to the limit on the exclusion.

The impact of the cap would depend on how employers and employees responded to the tax reform, but it is likely that there would be gradual and actually beneficial effects over time. One effect would be a long over- due rebalancing of compensation. In recent years, total compensation has grown quite strongly in the United States, while cash earnings have not. The reason for this, especially since 2000, has been that tax-free fringe ben- efits have risen as a proportion of total compensation. The present unlim- ited tax exclusion encourages this trend. A limit on the exclusion would encourage employees to consider accepting more of their compensation in other forms. Some might opt for more tax-advantaged education and retirement savings while many would opt for more cash income. Another long-term effect would be to encourage employees, not just employers, to press for more economical health services in the future.

CREATE A REFUNDABLE, ADVANCEABLE, AND ASSIGNABLE TAX CREDIT FOR LOWER-INCOME FAMILIES. Several lawmakers have put forward tax reform proposals designed to replace the current federal tax exclusion (in whole or in part) with a federal tax credit to help make health insurance

Ftn. 7 more affordable for lower-income families.[7] A credit is more efficient and more vertically equitable than a deduction or an exclusion. A credit also is more flexible and can be calibrated to concentrate most or all of the tax subsidy on lower-income families. Some proposals use simple credits while others (for example, Butler 2001) recommend more complex credits designed to address various goals, such as minimizing work disincentives and adapting the credit for families with severe medical needs.

The most practical form of tax credit for a lower-income family would cover most of the cost of a reasonable level of coverage in the family's geographic area while retaining the incentive to seek value for money. Families with incomes below 200 percent of the official family poverty level (which was approximately $21,200 for a family of four in 2008), for instance, could be made eligible for a federal tax credit to offset 90 percent of the cost of a health plan, capped at the average cost of major basic plans in the state. If an employee were offered coverage through the workplace, the employee could use the credit for that coverage only, and the credit would apply only to the out-of-pocket costs the employee incurs under the plan.

The structure, which is open to many variants, is intended to achieve certain important goals. One is to ensure that the credit covers most of a base insurance plan for lower-income families wherever they live. Analyses indicate that many are unwilling or feel unable to pay for a plan unless the net cost (including both out-of-pocket costs and premiums) is close to zero (Sheils and Haught 2003, pp. A6–A8). A second goal is to balance costs and work incentives. A dilemma with credits and other subsidies is whether to phase them out rapidly as income rises, in which case the effective marginal tax rate can be very high and work is discouraged, or gradually, in which case the budget cost is very high as less-needy families are subsidized. This proposal envisions ending the credit abruptly once income eligibility is exceeded, to keep the arrangement simple and costs down. Such "cliff" approaches exist today in several major programs, such as Medicaid and the State Children's Health Insurance Program, and the negative impact on work is acceptable. A third goal is to prevent tax "double-dipping." Since workers with employer-sponsored coverage already receive an exclusion, the credit is limited to out-of-pocket insurance costs.

7. An example is the Tax Equity and Affordability Act (S. 3754), introduced in 2006 by Senator Mel Martinez (R-Fla.). A bill proposing a comprehensive restructuring of the tax treatment of health care, replacing the entire tax exclusion with a refundable tax credit, was introduced in 1993 (S. 1743, H.R. 3689) by Senator Don Nickles (R-Okla.) and Representative Cliff Stearns (R-Fla.).

The credits in the Health Exchange Plan would be refundable, advance-able, and assignable. Since millions of lower-income families pay little or no federal income tax, a credit would have to be refundable in order to provide any assistance, such that families whose calculated credit exceeded their tax liability would receive the difference in cash from the government. Advanceability—meaning that the credit would be available through the year rather than only at the end of the tax year—is important because oth-erwise many lower-income families would likely be unable to pay their pre-miums when due. Such an advanceable credit could be factored into with-holding calculations at the place of work and into the proposed payroll deduction for premium payments. Finally, assignability means that the credit could be transferred from the individual to the chosen health plan in return for a reduced premium—much as in the FEHBP, where the govern-ment subsidy for the federal worker is paid directly to the plan and the pre-mium is correspondingly reduced. This is simple and particularly helpful for families who do not earn enough to have to fill out a tax return.

Possible Variations on the Basic Proposal

The three-part proposal outlined above contains several precisely specified features. But a number of variations in these features would also be com-patible with the broad goals.

Designing Insurance Exchanges: State and Federal Roles

The Health Exchange Plan views insurance exchanges as the most promis-ing vehicle to accomplish the goal of a state-based framework for insurance plans to achieve more effective pooling, better spreading of risk, and real portability. But the details of regulations to reach those goals are left to the states, on the grounds that they are best placed to develop rules for their particular situation and to experiment with new approaches.

To be sure, there are differences of opinion as to what the best state rules would be. While the Massachusetts legislation requires tight commu-nity rating (all persons in a given community pay the same premium), exchange proposals in Maryland and the District of Columbia permit rat-ing bands based on age and other criteria (Haislmaier and Owcharenko 2006, pp. 1584–85). States should experiment with alternative strategies for constructing large, stable pools for coverage through the exchanges. One possible way to stabilize a voluntary pool, for instance, is to charge lower premiums to those who remain insured within the pool than to those who move in and out of coverage. The proposals for Maryland and the

District of Columbia, for example, would allow insurers to impose premium surcharges and some restrictions on preexisting conditions on persons who have gaps in coverage (Haislmaier and Owcharenko 2006, p. 1585). In addition, states could encourage the offering of long-term insurance contracts.

To arrange stable and affordable coverage, states also need to experiment with ways to adjust for selection effects among plans within the pool. Age-related premium bands, for example, would make coverage more affordable for younger, healthier individuals, inducing those who are better risks to participate in the pool. States might also apply reinsurance or insurer "risk-transfer" pool requirements to all coverage sold within a state, whether inside or outside of the exchange. The Maryland and District of Columbia proposals would establish such a special "back-end" risk adjuster, with all insurers required to contribute to a common pool, from which payments would be made back to the insurers to adjust for disparities in enrollment levels of high-cost individuals.[8]

An insurance exchange would ensure true portability of insurance within a state for the families of workers who move between employers offering access to the exchange (assuming the insurance plan is available in their new neighborhood if they move within a state). To achieve portability across state lines, states might draw up agreements to link their exchanges and allow transfers between states.

A NATIONAL INSURANCE EXCHANGE? Some might argue that a national exchange, or set of national exchanges, would be better and more practical than state-level exchanges. To be sure, states do vary in their capacity to develop and implement innovative proposals such as health exchanges. But establishing a federal system of exchanges would not be a wise variant of the proposal.

For one thing, the regulation of insurance in the private sector is primarily a state function. Thus any attempt to create a national exchange or to introduce federally designed exchanges at the state level would immediately be sidetracked into a debate over the federal preemption of state insurance laws and the form and structure of the new federal regulations that would be applied to plans sold through a national exchange. Second,

---

8. Interestingly, the problem of adverse selection in the community-rated FEHBP is less severe than might be expected. A probable explanation, write Curtis Florence and Kenneth Thorpe (2003), is that the premium subsidy level for federal employees is sufficiently large that even though employees seek good value at the margin, many healthier employees still choose very comprehensive benefits.

those families who would benefit most from an exchange are typically those employed in small or medium-size firms in one geographic location, and a state-based reform design can more easily address local conditions. Third, although certain general characteristics of an exchange are essential if it is to achieve the goals of reform, there are many different ways to design the details to accommodate different local conditions. Finally, it is generally easier to get important changes under way with an evaluation or demonstration project on a smaller scale, which would yield valuable experience and evidence that might shape broader national reforms later. This does not mean that every state must be an innovator. As with most state-based innovations in public policy in other areas, such as welfare and education, certain states would likely take the lead in designing exchanges while others would tend to follow.

"OUTCOME-BASED" STATE RULES TO FOSTER COVERAGE THROUGH EXCHANGES. State-based rules for insurance exchanges could still be harmonized with national goals for reducing the number of uninsured without unduly restricting state flexibility and innovation. The proposed state-centered approach, for example, is compatible with proposals that would condition tax relief and federal health funding on plausible state action to make insurance available and affordable. The approach is also compatible with bills now before Congress that would encourage states to propose to the federal government a range of steps to reduce uninsurance within their borders, including congressionally enacted legislative waivers from existing federal laws and programs. These bills would provide waivers and federal grants for an experimental period, depending on how successful the state was in reaching agreed outcome measures.[9]

Employer and Individual Mandates

The Health Exchange Plan does not include a mandate on employers to participate in the exchange, but states could decide to include one (excluding ERISA-regulated employers choosing to retain their company plan). States could also decide whether or not to require employers to contribute

---

9. Bipartisan bills now before both houses would significantly change federal law and allow states to make significant changes in their laws to reduce uninsurance. Examples are the legislation (H.R. 506) introduced by Representatives Tammy Baldwin (D-Wisc.) and Tom Price (R-Ga.) and legislation (S. 325) by Senators George Voinovich (R-Ohio) and Jeff Bingaman (D-N.Mex.). For an analysis of this general approach, see Henry J. Aaron and Stuart M. Butler, "How Federalism Could Spur Bipartisan Action on the Uninsured," *Health Affairs*, web exclusive, March 31, 2004 (content.healthaffairs.org/cgi/reprint/hlthaff.w4.168v1.pdf).

to an employee's plan through an exchange, although such a requirement would surely be offset by reduced wage compensation.

It might be argued that the Health Exchange Plan would be more likely to reach the goal of universal coverage if it contained an individual or employer mandate (or both). To be sure, the proposal is compatible with the idea of individual or employer mandates and could operate smoothly if a state were to introduce such requirements. That would be up to the state, in keeping with the state-centered approach. But the proposal is designed to begin a gradual evolution of employer-based coverage with the active support of employers. An employer mandate risks triggering opposition from the key business constituency while perpetuating the myth that employers "pay for" coverage when the cost really comes out of total compensation.

A limited form of individual mandate can be justified as a way of enforcing appropriate personal responsibility in a society that underwrites emergency room care for the uninsured. Nevertheless, the proposal omits an individual mandate for two reasons. The first is that such a mandate is unfair unless the individual or family has the means to carry it out. Perhaps when all the tax reforms proposed above are fully implemented, all individuals and families could then afford coverage, and a mandate would be reasonable. But it might not work out that way. The second reason is that a controversial individual mandate might not in any case be needed to achieve near-universal coverage, as the combination of tax reform with automatic enrollment and payroll deductions likely would sharply increase the proportion of working families signing up for coverage.

Employers as Facilitators: Automatic Enrollment

The payroll adjustment system in the Health Exchange Plan might be enhanced by encouraging employers to adopt automatic enrollment. Although a mandate on employers to include automatic enrollment would be unwise and would likely trigger political opposition, states choosing to require firms to make the exchange available to their employees could include a requirement for automatic enrollment. Under this arrangement, employers would automatically withhold a premium from each employee sufficient for individual or family coverage under a "base option" plan designated by the state and available through the exchange. Employees could avoid this default enrollment by designating an alternative plan, much as workers can avoid an automatic tax withholding amount by indicating another amount on their W-4 form. Absent a state individual mandate to purchase basic insurance, under automatic enrollment employees could decline coverage altogether by signing a document indicating that they understood the consequences of lack of coverage.

The idea of automatic enrollment has been gaining interest in recent years as a means of increasing the take-up rate of health and savings plans at the workplace while increasing administrative efficiency.[10] The automatic enrollment system used for Part B premiums in Medicare achieves sign-up rates of over 90 percent. And evidence from workplace automatic enrollment for 401(k) plans suggests that it can sharply increase sign-up rates for insurance. Studies by Brigitte Madrian and others (Madrian and Shea 2000; Choi and others 2005), for instance, found that automatic enrollment boosted 401(k) enrollment from 13 percent to 80 percent among workers earning less than $20,000 a year.

Reforming the Tax Treatment of Health Insurance

DESIGNING A TAX CAP. The Health Exchange Plan includes a cap on the value of an insurance plan that can be excluded from taxable income, but this cap could be designed in a variety of ways, depending on economic, budget, and political considerations. The tax "bite" over time, and hence the revenue generated to finance a tax credit, would in part depend on the index used, if any, to adjust the cap each year, and this would depend on political feasibility. The proposal uses the CPI, whose rate of increase is well below average annual premium increases so that over time an increasing proportion of plans would exceed the cap. However, the revenue generated by a cap would also depend on the response of consumers and health care providers to the new limit on tax-advantaged insurance. If, as advocates of tax reform argue, the market responded with stronger competition and more cost consciousness on the part of consumers, the future rise in insurance premiums would be slower and new tax revenue would be less.

The proposal envisions that the "excess" coverage above the cap would be added to a family's taxable income, in the same way that excess contributions to an IRA or other limited tax-advantaged account are taxed, but only if family income exceeds a certain level. Initially an alternative approach might be to tax the excess only for those paying the alternative

10. For example, see Lynn Etheredge, "A Flexible Benefits Tax Credit for Health Insurance and More," *Health Affairs,* web exclusive, March 22, 2001 (content.health affairs.org/cgi/reprint/hlthaff.w1.1v1.pdf); Karen Davis and Cathy Schoen, "Creating Consensus on Coverage Choices," *Health Affairs,* web exclusive, April 23, 2003 (content. healthaffairs.org/cgi/reprint/hlthaff.w3.199v1.pdf); Jack Meyer and Sharon Silow-Carroll, "Building on the Job-Based Health Care System: What Would It Take?" *Health Affairs,* web exclusive, August 27, 2003 (content.healthaffairs.org/cgi/reprint/hlthaff.w3.415v1.pdf).

minimum tax. This income-based approach would avoid significant oppo-sition from (typically unionized) employees with very expensive health plans that constitute an unusually large proportion of their compensation. But making the excess taxable at all income levels would be an alternative and would raise more revenue to fund tax reform.

The revenue that the cap would yield over time could be used to enhance tax subsidies for the neediest working families. In his fiscal 2008 budget request, as noted above, President Bush proposed a cap of $7,500 in exclud-able health plans for individual workers ($15,000 for family coverage), although the revenue impact was complicated and blunted by offering a "standard deduction" equal to the cap for workers whose plans cost less.[11] In 2005 the Congressional Budget Office (CBO) examined the impact of a proposal to cap the personal tax exclusion for employer contributions to insurance and health accounts (such as flexible spending accounts) at $8,640 per year for family coverage and $3,720 for individuals. A cap at that level would affect most families with coverage, and the CBO estimated that it would yield $17.5 billion in revenue in 2006, rising to $59.9 billion in 2010 and $705.9 billion over 2006–15 (CBO 2005, p. 284).

Another version of a tax cap was introduced in 2006 by Senator Mel Martinez (R-Fla.). His bill (S. 3754) proposed to cap the tax exclusion at $5,000 for individual coverage and $11,500 for families. These amounts would not be indexed. According to Congress's Joint Committee on Taxa-tion, a cap at this level would have increased federal revenue by almost $24 billion in fiscal 2007, rising to over $68 billion in fiscal 2011. The committee estimated that this would cover more than four times the cost of a refundable tax credit for 100 percent of health insurance up to $2,000 for individuals and $4,000 for families if the credit were gradually phased down for family incomes above $30,000.[12] Capping the exclusion at the relatively low amounts in these examples would affect millions of Ameri-cans and so would be politically unwise, but they indicate how the impact grows over time. Capping at a much higher initial amount would be a wiser, more achievable step.

VARIETIES OF TAX CREDIT. Although the federal government would be responsible for most of the cost of a health insurance credit program, the states could be seen as partners in creating the credit, just as many other health programs are shared federal-state responsibilities. The proposed

11. For an analysis of the Bush proposal, see Burman and others (2007).
12. Letter to Senator Tom Coburn (R-Okla.) from Thomas Barthold, Deputy Chief of Staff, Joint Committee on Taxation, October 12, 2006.

reforms would benefit states financially by reducing the costs associated with uninsurance. Hence it would be reasonable to use some of those savings (such as the federal "disproportionate share" money for hospitals with many low-income and uninsured patients) to help cover the cost of the federal credit or to finance a state supplement to the federal subsidy. In addition, states with an income tax code mirroring the federal code would gain revenue from the cap on the tax exclusion, which could be used to supplement the credit.

The Health Exchange Plan envisions a credit that covers a percentage of the premium up to a maximum, with an income eligibility cap and an abrupt ending of eligibility above the cap. But there is legitimate debate about the best design of such a credit given the multiple goals of maximizing target efficiency, minimizing budgetary cost, and optimally aligning consumer incentives. Reasonable designs include flat dollar amounts (which could be made taxable and so related to income), sliding-scale credits based on income, and credits based on expenditure compared with income. Credits might also be grafted onto other general reforms of the tax treatment, such as that proposed by President Bush.

There are also various ways to address the concern that reconciling tax credit payments at the end of the tax year, as with other tax breaks, could lead to severe financial difficulties for lower-income families who have misestimated their withholding because their income has changed through the year. That could discourage these families from applying for an advance on their credit, and that in turn would make the credit less effective in covering their premiums. A rough-and-ready alternative would be to base the credit amount on the family's income in the previous year. In the case of very low-income employees, the assignability of the proposed credit could avoid the need for reconciliation.

Questions and Answers about the Health Exchange Plan

What Would Be the Advantages for the Typical Family of an Insurance Plan Obtained through an Exchange?

Employed families in exchange-sponsored plans would have the advantage of workplace administration, with the employer responsible for the bookkeeping functions of premium payment and tax adjustment, and many would receive an employer contribution to the premium cost. But unlike with typical employer-sponsored coverage today—even coverage through large employers—these families would gain tax-advantaged access to a large range of exchange-sponsored plans. The family could choose a plan that meets its preferences, working perhaps through a trusted agent such as a labor organization or church consortium. Families could also retain their plan when a worker in the family switched jobs among employers in the exchange system.

A positive by-product of families retaining their coverage between jobs, and thus perhaps for many years or even decades, is that insurance companies would have a stronger incentive to offer policies designed and priced for long-term coverage. Today most health insurance, including employment-based group insurance, is priced and designed more for the short term because working families typically change coverage often during their lives as they change jobs. But as more and more families retained their coverage through participation in an exchange, renewable long-term contracts would likely become more common, as they are in life insurance, and there would likely be an increased emphasis on preventive services. Indeed, with the prospect of a longer-term relationship between insurer and insured, and especially if a reinsurance or risk adjustment system were created within the state, insurers likely would be more willing to accept long-term contracts with limited premium variation as a requirement of doing business.

Would There Be Significant Changes for Employees in Large Firms?

No. For large self-insured employers there would be no change in the way employees obtain coverage unless the firm and its employees decided to switch to the exchange-based system. If the firm's plan is regulated under ERISA, the state could not require the employer to offer access to the exchange-sponsored plans. Its employees typically would continue to receive employer-sponsored health benefits. If they switched to another employer with sponsored insurance, they would, as today, come under a new plan, perhaps with different benefits and service providers. If they changed jobs and did not move to another large firm with sponsored insurance, however, they could become eligible for portable, continuous insurance from the exchange by signing up through their new employer (if that employer participates in the exchange) or on their own as individuals.

Other firms could continue to sponsor commercial group insurance if they wished and if state law allowed it. Again the employees would see no change in their benefit availability today, and if they moved to another employer that sponsored coverage, they would come under that employer's plan. But if they switched jobs to an employer that participated in an exchange, they could sign up for an exchange-sponsored plan and keep that plan from employer to employer going forward.

Still other employers, including many who currently sponsor coverage, could decide instead to participate in the exchange and take on the role of facilitator of their employees' benefits. In this case the employer's role would be to arrange for the collection of premiums and make tax withholding adjustments, much as many of these same employers do today for employee savings plans, and remit the money to the exchange. These employers could, if they chose, make a financial contribution to their employees' coverage as a fixed contribution or even as a defined benefit-like percentage of the premium cost of some maximum level of plan. The government's contribution as an employer in the FEHBP takes this hybrid form.

Employees in firms large and small could be affected by the tax reform proposals, however, depending on their income and the value of their employer-sponsored plan. They would have to review their compensation package in this case and perhaps choose to take any "excess" benefits in some other form of compensation. Lower-paid employees in employer-sponsored plans who are eligible for a tax credit would have to use it for their employer's plan.

Doesn't the Health Exchange Plan Risk Weakening the Employment-Based System or Even Causing It to Unravel?

No. On the contrary, it would actually strengthen the existing system by putting it on a sounder footing that is more compatible with underlying trends in employment, the strengths and weaknesses of employers as organizers of coverage, and the generally accepted goal of portable, affordable, and continuous coverage.

The successful parts of the current employer-sponsored system would be largely untouched, other than by the limits placed on today's open-ended tax exclusion. But the less successful parts would be strengthened and rationalized in a number of ways. For one thing, the exchanges and the facilitator role envisioned for most employers would bolster coverage among employees in smaller firms by playing to the strengths of these firms while relieving them of the burdensome complexity and financial risk of sponsoring coverage. For another, the new tax credit available to households for out-of-pocket coverage would also induce many families to sign up for offered dependent coverage that they currently decline as too costly.

The proposal also includes features that would appropriately protect employment-based coverage from the adverse selection or "crowding-out" pressures that typically accompany efforts to help the uninsured, such as expansions in Medicaid, the State Children's Health Insurance Program, and other forms of government-sponsored coverage. For example, the tax credit must be used for employment-based coverage if such coverage is offered, avoiding the concern that younger, healthier employees might leave an employer's insurance pool. Moreover, firms currently vulnerable to adverse selection or gyrating insurance premiums because of a changing workforce could gain greater stability by transitioning to coverage offered through an exchange.

Rather than Give Credits to Individuals, Why Not Give Tax Incentives to Employers to Expand Traditional Coverage?

Subsidizing employers, especially smaller employers, to sponsor coverage would not fix the many limitations of employer-sponsored coverage discussed above. Moreover, targeting such tax subsidies efficiently would be very difficult, leading to very high federal costs for each additional insured family at those firms where a significant proportion of the workforce already signs up for insurance. And trying to target an employer subsidy only to lower-income households would compromise privacy by requiring the employer to know the employee's household income.

How Would the Value of an Employer-Sponsored Plan Be Determined for Purposes of Calculating the Amount in Excess of the Tax-Exempt Limit?

Employees do not receive information on the premium value of their group insurance on their year-end W-2s, and in the case of self-insured employer plans, there is not even a premium amount to report. So how could the value of coverage be assessed and fairly allocated between healthier and sicker employees?

It is certainly more complicated to assess tax on noncash group insurance products than on cash income, but we do have experience in capping the tax-free status of group insurance in the case of employer-paid life insurance. Only the first $50,000 of such insurance is excludable from the employee's taxable compensation. The group premium amount for additional coverage appears on the W-2 and is taxable. In this case—as would be the case with health insurance—because the imputed premium amount for "excess" life insurance is group rated, younger employees (who could get cheaper individual coverage) would pay comparatively more tax for the same benefit.[13]

---

13. I am grateful to my colleague Edmund Haislmaier for his guidance on the issue of estimating the tax value of employer-sponsored insurance.

Determining a premium value for the self-insured and self-funded coverage common in very large companies is indeed an issue. A simple approach would be to use the existing rules for COBRA coverage, which employers already must make available to departing employees. Another issue concerns the often significant difference (similar to the case of life insurance) between the nominal value of the group coverage and the actuarial value based on the employee's medical risk. Again, this is probably best addressed under existing federal discrimination law, which places limits on the permissible variation of premiums and contributions for different classes of employees. But in those companies with collective bargaining contracts, another option might be for the union and management to assign values to certain classes of employees in the context of an overall compensation agreement. An additional point is that there are typically other tax-advantaged health accounts available at the workplace, such as flexible spending accounts, and so a concern is that limiting the tax-free status of insurance provided directly by employers could lead simply to employers and employees trying to avoid the tax cap by agreeing to shift insurance into other tax-free accounts. This might be addressed by applying an aggregate cap to all tax-free employment-based accounts.

What Types of Trusted-Agent Organizations Might Offer Plans through Exchanges?

The creation of insurance exchanges, together with official clarification that exchange-sponsored plans would convey the same tax relief as employer-sponsored plans, likely would encourage certain types of organizations to organize insurance.

UNIONS. One likely agent would be unions, not just as advisers for households comfortable with unions but also as sponsors of plans. Unions and labor-based mutual societies have a long history in this country and others of acting as "friendly societies" that offer benefits, not just as benefit negotiators. Unions are also active as health sponsors in other ways, for example, as organizers of plans under the Taft-Hartley Act. These plans are common in the construction industry but also are offered in other industries where employment is often interrupted or where workers frequently move between employers, such as in the hotel sector. Some unions also are already significant plan sponsors in the FEHBP, where many nonunion workers are able to pick coverage offered through unions. One of the largest plans, the Mail Handlers Benefit Plan, with over 250,000 enrollees, is not restricted to regular union members; indeed, the plan has five times as many enrollees as regular union members. Others join because the union has assembled an attractive set of benefits and acts as the agent for its enrollees.

RELIGIOUS ORGANIZATIONS. Health plans arranged by religious organizations would also become more widespread if members could obtain tax or other assistance to purchase coverage through these groups. American churches and other religious associations and lodges have a long history of providing social services for their congregations and operating hospital systems. Indeed, religious fraternal organizations, many of them church affiliated and many of these African American, were a major source of health insurance—sometimes as capitated health plans reminiscent of today's health maintenance organizations (HMOs)—in the first part of the twentieth century (Beito 2000, chapters 9 and 10). These later declined, not because the sponsors ceased to be trusted agents but because the unsubsidized plans were unable to compete with tax-subsidized employer-sponsored insurance and Medicaid. Tax neutrality would level the playing field. For lower-income African Americans especially, the church today is often a far more stable institution in the community than local small employers—and has a long history of engagement in education, housing, and other social services.

OTHER NONEMPLOYER AGENTS. Other affinity groups, such as state farm bureaus and professional associations, exist in part to negotiate health coverage for their members. But again, the current tax code does not encourage employees in most instances to choose these agents, even if they are more trusted than their employers. Reform would likely lead to a resurgence in plans offered by these groups.

An important aspect of all such agent relationships is that the organization does not typically shoulder the insurance risk itself. More typically, the organization assembles the group and negotiates with an insurance carrier to provide the insurance, receiving a fee from the insurer for performing marketing and some management functions. Farm bureau plans typically offer coverage designed for rural families yet underwritten through a separate insurer. The Mail Handlers Benefit Plan, for instance, is backed by the First Health Group. In each case the organization is performing an agency role, much as many employers do, although large employers also typically carry a significant part of the insurance risk.[14]

14. Many large interstate employers self-insure, meaning that they themselves hold the insurance risk, although some also purchase catastrophic insurance. Sometimes firms self-insure in order to gain greater freedom from state insurance rules by instead coming under federal ERISA regulation. Other (typically medium-size or smaller) firms purchase insurance for their employees, contributing to coverage and contracting with an insurance company.

OTHER EMPLOYERS AS AGENTS OF HEALTH CARE COVERAGE. In the future, another possible alternative to one's own employer as health coverage agent might be other employers. After all, it is common for large companies to sell to the public certain services initially designed for internal use. For example, after telecommunications deregulation in the 1960s and 1970s allowed other carriers to compete with AT&T's long-distance monopoly, some major firms decided to offer their internal communications services outside the firm.[15] The Southern Pacific Railroad, for instance, opened up its internal communications network to outside customers under the brand name Sprint. Other companies have taken advantage of relatively neutral tax laws and regulations in finance to offer services originally designed for their own operations. The General Motors Acceptance Corporation, for example, offers a wide range of insurance and mortgage products to a market well beyond GM's initial exclusive focus on its car purchasers.

Unfortunately, the tax laws governing health insurance, unlike those governing the tax treatment of mortgage loans, discourage GM and other firms from taking similar steps to market their health plans to a wider public. Still, some companies have edged into the field. In particular, John Deere created its own HMO in the early 1980s, mainly for its own employees, and then began to offer coverage to other employers and purchased health operations to serve its new market. The company's for-profit health division even offered coverage to individuals as a Medicare HMO and provided managed care Medicaid services in several states and to federal workers under the FEHBP. The health company was sold to United Healthcare in 2006. Marketing to the FEHBP, Medicare, and Medicaid was attractive to Deere because the subsidies in those programs are not restricted to employees of the company. Making the tax system more neutral might encourage other companies to consider opening up their plans through insurance exchanges.

Could the First Two Elements of the Health Exchange Plan Proceed without the Tax Reform Element?

Yes. States and the federal government could move forward with insurance exchanges and the facilitator role for employers without restructuring the tax treatment of health insurance. If states, within current federal law, created exchanges similar to the Massachusetts Connector, families enrolling in exchange-sponsored plans via their employer would be eligible for

15. For a summary of these decisions, see Crandall and Ellig (1995, pp. 18–19).

today's tax exclusion. An explicit ruling or change in the law would help encourage states to create exchanges by clarifying policy and perhaps making it more flexible, but such a proviso would not be essential. The proposed structural tax reform would significantly improve the affordability of coverage for lower-income Americans and take advantage of the other elements in the proposal, but it is not a precondition for these other elements.

Could the Tax Reform Element Proceed without the First Two Elements?

Yes, but its impact would be greatly enhanced by the exchanges and the revised employer role. Reforming the tax treatment of health insurance alone certainly would result in a more equitable distribution of tax subsidies and greater coverage. But the impact of tax reform would be increased significantly by the other elements of the proposal—which is why they are central to it. The availability of the proposed tax credits within a state could be made conditional on whether the state takes active steps to make coverage more affordable and available, if not through the steps proposed here to enhance employment-based insurance, then through other state proposals designed to move toward universal coverage.

Conclusion

America's health insurance system for working families is completely out of step with the needs of today's mobile workforce. Millions of working families have no coverage at all, and those with employer-sponsored insurance face gaps in coverage and the loss of vital services whenever they change jobs or their work situation. Unlike the other intensely personal and important decisions a family makes, such as where to live and where to educate the children, access to the health care system for most working Americans is controlled by their employer, not by the family itself. And while government provides over $200 billion each year in tax relief to subsidize this system, most of that subsidy goes to those who need help the least while more needy working families get little or no assistance.

There are really two worlds in employer-sponsored insurance. There is the world of large firms, where coverage is broadly available and continuous—provided an employee remains working for that large firm. And there is the world of small firms, where employees face the enormous medical and economic insecurity of gaps in coverage.

It is time to recast this system, created almost accidentally in the context of the industrial era, into a system appropriate for the postindustrial world of a surging services sector, high labor mobility, and changing work arrangements. The key is to delink the availability, control, and subsidization of health coverage from the place of work. Those families and their employers who are satisfied with the current system could keep things the way they are. But those who are dissatisfied could join an alternative that has been allowed to evolve out of the traditional notion of employer-sponsored insurance. In the proposed new system, families could choose their coverage and keep it from job to job, thanks to state-based insurance exchanges and to employers willing to help manage the insurance transaction rather than sponsor insurance itself. Furthermore, the tax subsidy would be based on need. By slowly transforming today's health insurance system in this way, we would achieve greater economic as well as health security for America's working families.

References

Antos, Joseph. 2006. "Is There a Right Way to Promote Health Insurance through the Tax System?" AEI Working Paper 127. Washington: American Enterprise Institute (June 9).

Antos, Joseph, and Alice Rivlin, eds. 2007. *Restoring Fiscal Sanity 2007: The Health Spending Challenge.* Brookings.

Beito, David. 2000. *From Mutual Aid to Welfare.* University of North Carolina.

Burman, Len, and others. 2007. "An Evaluation of the President's Health Insurance Proposal." *Tax Notes* 114, no. 10: 1013–28.

Butler, Stuart M. 2001. "Reforming the Tax Treatment of Health Care to Achieve Universal Coverage." In *Covering America: Real Remedies for the Uninsured,* edited by Eliot K. Wicks, pp. 23–42. Washington: Economic and Social Research Institute.

Choi, James J., and others. 2005. "Optimal Defaults and Active Decisions." Working Paper 11074. Cambridge, Mass.: National Bureau of Economic Research (January).

Clemens-Cope, Lisa, Bowen Garrett, and Catherine Hoffman. 2006. "Changes in Employees' Health Insurance Coverage, 2001-2005." Issue paper. Washington: Kaiser Family Foundation.

Congressional Budget Office (CBO). 2005. *Budget Options.*

Crandall, Robert, and Jerry Ellig. 1995. *Economic Deregulation and Customer Choice: Lessons for the Electric Industry.* George Mason University, Center for Market Processes.

DeNavas-Walt, Carmen, Bernadette D. Proctor, and Cheryl Lee Hill. 2006. "Income, Poverty, and Health Insurance Coverage in the United States: 2005." Current Population Reports P60-231. U.S. Census Bureau (August).

Florence, Curtis S., and Kenneth E. Thorpe. 2003. "How Does the Employer Contribution for the Federal Employee Health Benefits Program Influence Plan Selection?" *Health Affairs* 22, no. 2: 211–18.

Fronstin, Paul. 2003. "Sources of Health Insurance and the Characteristics of the Uninsured: Analysis of the March 2003 Current Population Survey." Issue Brief 264. Washington: Employee Benefit Research Institute.

———. 2005. "Sources of Health Insurance and the Characteristics of the Uninsured: Analysis of the March 2005 Current Population Survey." Issue Brief 287. Washington: Employee Benefit Research Institute.

———. 2006. "Sources of Health Insurance and the Characteristics of the Uninsured: Analysis of the March 2006 Current Population Survey." Issue Brief 298. Washington: Employee Benefit Research Institute.

Furman, Jason. 2007. "The Promise of Progressive Cost Consciousness in Health-Care Reform." Discussion Paper 2007-05. Hamilton Project, Brookings.

Glied, Sherry A., and Phyllis C. Borzi. 2004. "The Current State of Employment-Based Health Coverage." *Journal of Law, Medicine and Ethics* 32, no. 3: 404–09.

Goodman, John C. 2006. "Employer-Sponsored, Personal, and Portable Health Insurance." *Health Affairs* 25, no. 6: 1556–66.

Haislmaier, Edmund F., and Nina Owcharenko. 2006. "The Massachusetts Approach: A New Way to Restructure State Health Insurance Markets and Public Programs." *Health Affairs* 25, no. 6: 1580–90.

Kaiser Family Foundation and Health Research and Education Trust. 2006. *Employer Health Benefits. 2006 Annual Survey.* Menlo Park, Calif., and Chicago.

Madrian, Brigitte C., and Dennis F. Shea. 2000. "The Power of Suggestion: Inertia in 401(k) Participation and Savings Behavior." Working Paper 7682. Cambridge, Mass.: National Bureau of Economic Research (May).

Selden, Thomas M., and Bradley M. Gray. 2006. "Tax Subsidies for Employment-Related Health Insurance: Estimates for 2006." *Health Affairs* 25, no. 6: 1568–79.

Sheils, John, and Randall Haught. 2003. "Appendix A: The Health Benefits Simulation Model: Uniform Methodology and Assumptions." In *Cost and Coverage Analysis of Ten Proposals to Expand Health Insurance Coverage.* Washington: Economic and Social Research Institute.

Singer, Sara J., Alan M. Garber, and Alain C. Enthoven. 2001. "Near-Universal Coverage through Health Plan Competition: An Insurance Exchange Approach." In *Covering America: Real Remedies for the Uninsured,* edited by Elliot K. Wicks, pp. 155–71. Washington: Economic and Social Research Institute.

U.S. Department of Labor. 2006. *America's Dynamic Workforce.* Government Printing Office.

U.S. House of Representatives. Committee on the Budget. 2004. "Statement of C. Eugene Steuerle, Senior Fellow, Urban Institute." 108 Cong. 2 sess. (October 6).

Whitmore, Heidi, and others. 2006. "Employers' Views on Incremental Measures to Expand Health Coverage." *Health Affairs* 25, no. 6: 1668–78.

A Comprehensive Cure

The Guaranteed Health Care Access Plan—A Voucher-Style Reform

4

EZEKIEL J. EMANUEL AND VICTOR R. FUCHS

The American health care system is a dysfunctional mess; its problems are well known. There are coverage problems: tens of millions are uninsured, others have poor coverage, and millions receive Medicaid, which looks comprehensive on paper but, because of extremely low reimbursement, is served by few providers. In addition, as costs rise, there has been—and will continue to be—a steady drop in employer-based insurance. There are cost problems: over the last thirty years, the rise in health care costs has exceeded the economy's rate of growth by 2.1 percentage points each year (Catlin and others 2008; Kaiser Family Foundation 2006).[1] The Congressional Budget Office predicts that health care will consume one of every five dollars of output in the entire economy by 2017.[2] Medicare is going bankrupt, and given present trends, it will consume all taxes collected under current law in slightly more than fifty years (Boards of Trustees 2007).

The opinions expressed are the authors' own. They do not represent any position or policy of the National Institutes of Health, the U.S. Public Health Service, or the U.S. Department of Health and Human Services.

1. See also Congressional Budget Office, "Technological Change and the Growth of Health Care Spending" (www.cbo.gov/ftpdocs/89xx/doc8947/toc.htm).

2. Centers for Medicare and Medicaid Services, "National Health Expenditure Projections, 2006–2016" (www.cms.hhs.gov/NationalHealthExpendData/downloads/proj2006. pdf); Congressional Budget Office, "The Budget and Economic Outlook: Fiscal Years 2008 to 2017" (www.cbo.gov/ftpdoc.cfm?index=7731).

There are serious quality problems: it has become part of the conventional wisdom that 100,000 Americans die each year from preventable medical errors; that only 55 percent of proven effective therapies are administered to adult patients who need them, and only 46 percent of proven effective therapies are administered to children who need them; and that fewer than 25 percent of doctors and hospitals have installed electronic medical records, despite their advantages for quality and efficiency (Kohn, Corrigan, and Donaldson 2000; McGlynn and others 2003; Mangione-Smith and others 2007; Wachter and Shojania 2004). Paradoxically, the huge amount of money the United States is currently spending on health care should be sufficient to provide high-quality care for all Americans.

Myriad reforms of the health care system have been proposed; they can be grouped into three broad categories (Fuchs and Emanuel 2005). First are incremental reforms, such as expanding the existing State Children's Health Insurance Program (SCHIP) to cover all uninsured children, expanding Medicare to cover people between fifty-five and sixty-five, installing electronic medical records in all physician offices and hospitals, or providing tax breaks to individuals to buy health coverage (Pauly 2001; Palmisano, Emmons, and Wozniak 2004; and Butler 2001). These reforms do not try to solve any single problem entirely, much less seek to change the fundamental structure of the health care system. Rather they try to make headway mainly by expanding coverage.

Second are individual and employer mandates. While employer mandates have long been proposed—frequently under the title of "pay or play"—individual mandates are the health reform of the moment, having been enacted in Massachusetts and proposed in California and Pennsylvania (Gruber 2006). Mandates are a "fill-in-the-cracks" approach that aims for nearly 100 percent coverage by requiring that individuals or employers or both buy insurance. To enable them to do so, these plans typically expand Medicaid, create new insurance exchanges such as Massachusetts's Health Care Connector, and provide income-linked or other subsidies so that all can afford health insurance (Enthoven and Kronick 1989). These mandates aim at extending coverage, but they keep the current health care financing and delivery systems largely in place. Consequently, the problems of cost and quality are largely ignored.

Single-payer plans have long been proposed (Physicians' Working Group 2003; Krugman and Wells 2006).[3] "Single payer" is a capacious term that

---

3. Paul Krugman and Robin Wells, "The Health Care Crisis and What to Do about It," *New York Review of Books*, March 23, 2006.

could refer to any plan that relies on tax revenue to finance health care, but in the U.S. context, the term is associated with a distinctive approach to reform modeled on Medicare or on the Canadian health care system. Advocates of a single-payer plan would establish a single national health plan; eliminate private insurance and for-profit providers; create a national drug formulary, negotiating reduced drug and device costs; and use the expected large savings from reduced insurance underwriting, sales, and marketing costs as well as savings on drug costs to achieve universal coverage and expand the range of services provided. Most of the single-payer plans currently proposed enshrine fee-for-service payment for physicians and hospitals with a national fee schedule. Some more radical versions go further and call for negotiated operating budgets with hospitals with strict limits on capital expenditures (Physicians' Working Group 2003).

Although incremental reforms, mandates, and single-payer plans all address some of the key problems of the American health care system, all have important operational and political flaws (Fuchs and Emanuel 2005; Emanuel 2008). To a significant extent, all of these reforms focus on the financing of care and none tries to establish financial incentives that significantly improve the delivery of care. To address the problems of coverage, cost, and quality in a sustainable, feasible manner, we offer a fourth alternative: the Guaranteed Health Care Access Plan, a voucher-based reform (Emanuel 2008). But before considering this alternative, it is worth asking what, if anything, can be learned from these other proposals.

It is hard to see what can be learned from proposals for incremental reform. These proposals would not achieve universal coverage, would increase rather than decrease health care expenditures, and would leave the current dysfunctional financing and delivery systems essentially unchanged.

Individual and employer mandates stress the value of the insurance exchange. If we as a nation decide to retain private health care delivery by health plans and insurance companies, then using such arrangements to create extremely large purchasing pools can significantly reduce insurance underwriting, sales, and marketing costs. Insurance exchanges can also permit community rating, in which the premiums charged are the same for everyone while the payments to insurance companies are risk adjusted to minimize adverse selection. But *voluntary* exchanges are inherently unstable. As the experience of the now defunct PacAdvantage in California and other voluntary insurance exchanges has shown, they lead to adverse selection. If employers or individuals can opt in or out of the insurance exchange, the enrollees tend to be disproportionately the sicker patients whose higher costs set off a vicious cycle of ever-higher premiums and reductions in enrollment.[4] This suggests that any sustainable insurance exchange system needs to have *mandatory* enrollment and risk adjustment of payments so that an insurance company will be fairly compensated if its average enrollees are in particularly poor health. Moreover, because mandates by themselves do not fundamentally change the health care delivery system, they can do little to stem long-term cost increases or improve quality of care.

Advocates of single-payer plans argue that a central financing mechanism can achieve tremendous administrative savings and, by removing employers from the business of providing health insurance for their employees, can generate substantial labor efficiencies, thus stimulating the economy. This is true. However, creating a tax-financed system permits one-time savings—it does not affect the rate of increase in health care costs over time. Lowering the steep slope of the upward curve of health care spending can only be achieved by changing the delivery system to provide incentives, information, and infrastructure for more integrated and cost-effective delivery of care. Such changes in the delivery system are impossible within a single-payer system focused on minimizing administrative and drug costs while leaving the fee-for-service reimbursement system in place.

The Essential Elements of the Guaranteed Health Care Access Plan

How can we integrate central financing of health care with large purchasing pools to gain the advantages of single-payer plans and mandates while avoiding their disadvantages? We propose the Guaranteed Health Care Access Plan, a voucher-based reform, as the comprehensive cure for the ailing American health care system (Emanuel and Fuchs 2005; Emanuel 2008). The Guaranteed Health Care Access Plan involves a ten-step therapy (see table 4-1).

Guaranteed Health Care for All Americans

All U.S. residents would receive a health care certificate or voucher good for the acquisition of health coverage through a qualified health plan or insurance company. At first, those who currently receive coverage through Medicare, Medicaid, SCHIP, or another government program would choose whether to stay with their current program or join the voucher

---

4. PacAdvantage, "PacAdvantage Will No Longer Provide Access to Health Insurance Offerings," press release, August 11, 2006 (www.pacadvantage.org/documents/brokers/Final_PA_News_Release.pdf).

Table 4-1. Ten Main Features of the Proposed Guaranteed Health Care Access Plan

Feature	Description
Guaranteed health care for all	Each household would receive a voucher for coverage through a qualified health plan or insurance company. The voucher would not be a cash voucher denominated in dollars to buy health services but rather would be an insurance voucher entitling the holder to enrollment in a health plan of the holder's choice. There would be no premiums or deductibles and minimal copayments to remove financial barriers to health insurance. Qualified plans must accept the voucher for the standard benefits package. Plans would be reimbursed a risk-adjusted premium for enrollees.
Standard health benefits	Standard benefits would be generous, modeled on services currently received by members of Congress and other federal employees through the Federal Employees Health Benefits program.
Freedom of choice	Americans would be able to choose from among several health plans. Plans would be required to accept any enrollee without exclusions for preexisting conditions and with guaranteed renewability.
Freedom to purchase additional services	Americans could choose to buy, with after-tax dollars, additional services and amenities such as wider selection of physicians and hospitals, coverage of complementary medicines, additional mental health benefits, or even "concierge medicine."
Funding through a dedicated value-added tax (VAT)	Financing for the vouchers would come from a dedicated VAT of about 10 to 12 percent on purchases of goods and services (to cover Americans not in Medicare or Medicaid). Revenue from the tax could not be diverted to other uses such as defense or Social Security. Congress could raise the VAT rate to cover more services.
End of employer-based insurance	The tax exemption for employer-based health insurance would be eliminated. Employers would probably stop offering health insurance, and current wages would rise in line with what employers contribute to health insurance premiums.
Phasing out of Medicare, Medicaid, SCHIP, and other government health programs	No one receiving benefits from Medicare, Medicaid, SCHIP, or any other government program would be forced out, but there would be no new enrollees. Current enrollees would have the option of joining the Guaranteed Health Care Access Plan. Over about ten to fifteen years these programs would shrink in size and eventually disappear.
Independent oversight	A National Health Board and twelve regional health boards would be created on the model of the Federal Reserve System. Members of the National Board and regional boards would be nominated by the president and confirmed by the Senate for long, staggered terms (for example, ten years). Dedicated funding would make the boards independent of annual congressional appropriations and help insulate them from political lobbying. The National Board would define and adjust the standard benefits, conduct research on risk adjustment, determine quality indicators, and report to the public about the health care system. The regional boards would certify insurance companies; establish and oversee insurance exchanges, enrollment in insurance companies, and payment to insurance companies; and collect and disseminate data on quality of care provided by insurance companies.
Cost and quality control measures	A new Institute for Technology and Outcomes Assessment would assess the effectiveness and cost of new drugs, medical devices, diagnostic tests, and other interventions on the basis of both existing research and new studies commissioned by the institute. The institute would also assess the outcomes of patients in the different health plans. Results of the assessments would be publicly disseminated in ways that protect patient confidentiality. To ensure objectivity and independence, the institute would be funded by a dedicated share of the VAT revenue, estimated at 0.5 percent.

(*continued*)

Table 4-1. Ten Main Features of the Proposed Guaranteed Health Care Access Plan (*Continued*)

Feature	Description
Patient safety and dispute resolution measures	Each regional health board would create a regional Center for Patient Safety and Dispute Resolution to receive and evaluate claims of injury by patients, compensate those patients found to have been injured by medical error, and, when appropriate, discipline or disqualify from practice physicians who repeatedly provide poor quality care. The regional centers would also evaluate interventions to enhance patient safety and would coordinate and fund implementation of valuable interventions by health plans, hospitals, physicians, and others. Physicians would likely pay greatly reduced premiums to cover those (probably rare) malpractice awards in cases that go to court. The centers would be funded by a dedicated 2.5 percent of the VAT revenue.

system. Unlike a health savings account, the health care certificate would not provide a specified dollar amount to be used to buy individual medical services over the year but instead would convey the right to enroll in a health plan that covers a set of standard benefits. In other words, it would be an insurance voucher, not a cash voucher. The recipient would pay nothing directly for the health care certificate itself or for the benefits that it covers; financing would be accomplished through a dedicated value-added tax (VAT) described below. There would be no deductibles and minimal copayments.

Regional health boards would certify that each health plan and insurance company has a sufficient network of hospitals and physicians and adequate financial reserves, and that the plan or company is in fact providing the standard benefits. To participate in the Guaranteed Health Care Access Plan, health plans and insurance companies would have to guarantee enrollment and renewability every year for all applicants without consideration of their medical history: they could not turn anyone away for any reason, would have to guarantee renewability, and could not refuse to cover preexisting conditions. The regional boards would pay each plan and company a risk-adjusted premium for each person or family enrolled. To minimize the financial incentive for plans and companies to cherry-pick the healthiest patients and avoid enrolling sicker ones, the regional health boards would adjust the premium for age, sex, smoking status, preexisting conditions, and other factors.

Standard Benefits

The health care certificate would cover a set of comprehensive benefits modeled on the generous benefits that federal employees, including members of Congress, receive today through the Federal Employees Health Benefits (FEHB) program.[5] These benefits include coverage for preventative screenings, brand name and generic prescription drugs, dental care, home and office visits, hospitalization, physical and occupational therapy, and mental health inpatient and outpatient care. The plan also allows patients to choose their own doctors and hospitals, requires no referral for specialist visits, and charges low copayments. To qualify for participation in the Guaranteed Health Care Access Plan, health plans and insurance companies would have to agree to provide these standard benefits for the value of the health care certificate. Those that qualify, however, would otherwise be free, for the most part, to structure their businesses as they see fit. They could shrink (within limits) or expand their physician and hospital networks. They could offer different drug formularies, more disease management programs, or a larger or smaller choice of specialists or specialty hospitals, or make other modifications. They could even offer, at an additional charge, benefits not part of the standard benefits. But, other than copayments, they could not charge enrollees for coverage of the standard benefits.

The health plans and insurance companies would have to provide aggregate data on their own past performance, including patient satisfaction, disenrollment rates, hospitalization and mortality rates for various conditions (such as diabetes, emphysema, and heart attacks), patient outcomes for various conditions, and other quality measures.

Freedom of Choice

Like today's programs with mandates, the Guaranteed Health Care Access Plan would establish an insurance exchange in each region of the country to facilitate enrollment by individuals and families in the health care plan of their choice. All Americans except those who prefer to remain in Medicare, Medicaid, or SCHIP would receive their coverage by enrolling through the insurance exchange. Participating health plans and insurance companies would be private and would not be run by the government. In most regions, consumers would have freedom of choice among several qualified health plans or insurance companies—probably five to eight but as many as twenty or more in some locales. They would be free to change plans each year or to select a three-year enrollment option that would provide them with some additional benefits. Americans who fail to enroll themselves in a health plan or insurance program would be assigned to one, on an equitable basis, by the exchange in their region.

5. For a full set of FEHB benefits, see Blue Cross–Blue Shield, "Federal Employee Program Service Benefit Plan: 2007 Benefits" (www.fepblue.org/benefits/benefits07/benftaagso-07.html).

Freedom to Purchase Additional Services

Individuals and families would be free to purchase additional health care services or amenities that are not part of the standard health benefits. These might include greater choice of physicians and hospitals, access to a wider range of drugs or more brand name drugs, wider choice of eyeglasses, more mental health benefits, or even a "concierge medicine" package that eliminates time limits on office visits and provides for physicians to make house calls. However, payments for this additional coverage would not be tax deductible; they would be paid for with after-tax dollars, as is the case for food, clothing, and other consumer goods.

Funding by a Dedicated VAT

Funding for the vouchers would come entirely from a dedicated value-added tax, similar to a sales tax on purchases of goods and services. Initially, without Medicare and Medicaid beneficiaries, the VAT would be about 10 to 12 percent on all purchases subject to the tax. All the money raised, and only that money, would be used to support the voucher system. Thus there would be a direct connection between the VAT rate and the level of services included in the core benefits—the more generous the benefits, the higher the tax rate would have to be. Congress would have the power to set and adjust the VAT rate.

An End to Employer-Based Insurance

The current tax benefit for employer-based health insurance would be eliminated. Since under the Guaranteed Health Care Access Plan all workers would receive health care certificates for the standard health benefits, they would no longer look to their employers for health insurance. Workers would likely demand higher wages instead. Employer competition for workers would push up wages in those firms that previously provided insurance. (If it is legal, it might be possible to require employers to increase the wages of workers by the amount previously paid for the employer-based health insurance premium.) Some employers might still provide extended coverage for health care services not included in the standard benefits as a fringe benefit to attract or reward workers. This could be done in either of two ways: the employer could offer a specific dollar amount to its workers to pay for certain noncovered services (a defined contribution), or the employer could purchase an insurance plan on the workers' behalf. In either case, these added benefits would be taxed like other compensation rather than being exempt from tax as employer-provided health benefits are today.

Phasing Out of Medicare, Medicaid, SCHIP, and Other Government Health Insurance Programs

Americans whose health care is currently paid through Medicare, Medicaid, SCHIP, or another government health insurance program would not be forced to switch to the Guaranteed Health Care Access Plan. Initially, the Guaranteed Health Care Access Plan would cover the 220 million Americans who are not insured through Medicare, Medicaid, SCHIP, or other means-tested government programs. The remaining 80 million Americans who are enrolled in these government programs (Kaiser Family Foundation 2006) would have the choice of remaining in their government-funded program or joining the Guaranteed Health Care Access Plan. However, there would be no new enrollees in Medicare, Medicaid, SCHIP, or other current programs. Americans who turn sixty-five after the Guaranteed Health Care Access Plan goes into effect would remain in the new system. Similarly, those now receiving Medicaid or SCHIP would have to switch permanently to the Guaranteed Health Care Access Plan if they get a job or otherwise become ineligible for their current program. Thus, over time, fewer and fewer people would participate in these government-run health programs. Within essentially fifteen years, all Americans would receive the same standard benefits within the same health care delivery system. There would be one universal health care system—a public guarantee with private provision of services—for all Americans regardless of age, income, employment, health, or marital status.

Independent Oversight

To reduce political interference and allow tough administrative choices to be made, a National Health Board and twelve regional health boards would be established, modeled on the Federal Reserve System. Members of the National Health Board and the regional health boards would be nominated by the president and confirmed by the Senate for a long fixed term (say, ten years), which could be renewed only once. The terms of the board members would be staggered, with the term of only one member expiring in any given year.

The administrative budgets of the National Health Board and the regional health boards would be funded from the dedicated VAT, not by an annual appropriation by Congress. The National Health Board would have responsibility to

—define and regularly adjust the standard health benefits to reflect changes in standards of care, advances in technology, and fiscal realities;

—conduct research to determine the risk adjustments necessary for the premiums paid to health plans;

—determine payment differences based on geography;

—sponsor research on quality, outcomes, and performance of the health care system;

—oversee and coordinate the regional health boards; and

—report regularly to Congress and the American public on the health care system.

Within their geographic regions, the twelve regional health boards would have responsibility to

—certify and oversee the participating health plans and insurance companies and ensure that they have sufficient financial reserves and medical resources to provide the health services offered in the standard benefits package;

—oversee the insurance exchanges;

—manage the enrollment of individuals and families in health plans and insurance companies and assign to a health plan those who do not enroll on their own;

—pay the health plans and insurance companies the risk-adjusted premiums on their enrollees' behalf; and

—collect, analyze, and disseminate information on the quality of health care delivered by the individual health plans and insurance companies.

Cost and Quality Control Mechanisms

An Institute for Technology and Outcomes Assessment would be created to judge the value of new drugs, medical devices, diagnostic tests, and other medical interventions and to assess patient outcomes under the system. This institute would be responsible for

—systematic review of research studies and other data on the effectiveness, clinical effectiveness, and cost of different drugs, devices, diagnostic tests, and other interventions;

—commissioning of research studies to compare the clinical effectiveness of drugs, devices, diagnostic tests, and other interventions;

—collecting data from health plans and insurance companies on patient outcomes and on the drugs, devices, diagnostic tests, and interventions used; and

—disseminating data on technology and outcomes assessments to health plans, physicians, patients, drug and technology manufacturers, and the general public, while respecting patient confidentiality.

To ensure the independence and objectivity of the institute's work, funding would come from a fixed share (estimated at 0.5 percent) of the total revenues of the dedicated VAT. In addition, its operations would be overseen by an independent board appointed by the National Health Board.

Centers for Patient Safety and Dispute Resolution

Each regional health board would create a regional Center for Patient Safety and Dispute Resolution. These centers would be responsible for

—receipt and adjudication of patient complaints about medical errors and injuries;

—compensation of patients where it is found that their injuries were caused by medical error;

—discipline and disqualification from practice of physicians and other health professionals who repeatedly injure patients or violate established safety procedures;

—development of programs to promote patient safety; and

—coordination with health plans, hospitals, physicians, visiting nurses, and others to implement interventions proven to enhance patient safety.

Patients who believe they have been injured and are not satisfied by the center's resolution of their complaint would still be able to sue for malpractice.

Funding for the centers and for compensation to injured patients would come from the dedicated VAT. Since the current malpractice system costs about $20 billion a year (Congressional Budget Office 2004), approximately 2.5 percent of the VAT's total revenues would be required. With the centers paying for initial investigation, adjudication, and compensation, physicians would not have to pay malpractice premiums. They could still retain minimal insurance in case patients are dissatisfied with the resolution by the centers and elect to sue, but only a small amount of insurance should be necessary.

Economics of the Guaranteed Health Care Access Plan

We believe that any comprehensive health care reform proposal should meet two basic criteria. First, current national health expenditures should not have to increase to cover all Americans. That is, the initial cost of the Guaranteed Health Care Access Plan should not exceed the amount being spent on health care at this time. The health care system does not need more money—it needs to spend the money more efficiently. Second, the rate of increase in health care spending over time should reflect the growth of the economy and the public's willingness and ability to pay for health care services.

Would instituting the Guaranteed Health Care Access Plan increase or decrease national health care costs at the time it is instituted? In 2006, the annual premium for the FEHB program varied by state, but the premium in the high-end Blue Cross–Blue Shield preferred provider plan that serves as the basis for the voucher system's proposed standard benefit was $5,174 for individuals and $11,216 for families. Table 4-2 indicates that the total cost (using the 2006 premiums) for all 258 million Americans except those in Medicare would be $944 billion.

Many who are currently uninsured are young, healthy individuals—self-defined "invincibles"—who choose not to insure themselves. But others are uninsured because they are unhealthy and cannot obtain insurance, or have low incomes and cannot afford it, or both. The Medicaid population tends to be sicker than the federal employee population, and therefore they use more health care services and their costs are likely to be higher. A study by the Urban Institute estimates that, for an equivalent level of coverage, the uninsured and Medicaid populations incur about 26 percent higher costs per person than employed populations with private insurance (Holahan, Bovbjerg, and Hadley 2006). The uninsured and Medicaid populations under age sixty-five account for about 25 percent of the total U.S. population under age sixty-five. Costs under the voucher system would therefore be $61.4 billion higher than the $944 billion calculated based on premium rates for the FEHB program. This increase raises the total estimate to $1,005.6 billion.

This is a large sum, but it needs to be compared with current health spending for the same population. In 2006 (the most recent year for which data are available), federal and state governments spent $269 billion on Medicaid, excluding what they spent on nursing home care. In 2006 the total expenditure for private health insurance was $723 billion; this figure excludes out-of-pocket expenses for prescriptions, dental services, and other products (Catlin and others 2008). In addition, more than $10 billion a year is spent on additional safety net programs, such as maternal and child health programs, and hospital construction that would no longer be needed under the Guaranteed Health Care Access Plan. These expenditures sum to $1,002 billion (in 2006 dollars) for the 258 million Americans not currently receiving Medicare. This means that the Guaranteed Health Care Access Plan would not increase total national expendi-

Table 4-2. Projected Costs of the Proposed Guaranteed Health Care Access Plan versus Current System Costs

Units as indicated

Health care system	Number (millions)	Average annual premium (2006 dollars)	Total annual costs (billions of 2006 dollars)
Guaranteed Health Care Access Plan[a]			
Group served			
Individuals	41.2	5,174	213.2
Families	65.2[b]	11,216	731.3
Total non-Medicare population	257.6	. . .	944.5
Increase for extra use by uninsured and Medicaid populations	25 percent of population	Added costs per person: 26 percent more than the average	61.4
Total non-Medicare	257.6	. . .	1,005.9[c]
Current employer-based system[d]			
Type of insurance			
Medicaid	. . .	. . .	269[e]
Private health insurance	. . .	. . .	723
Other	. . .	. . .	10
Total non-Medicare			1,002

Source: Authors' calculations.

a. 2006 rates and expenditures. Annual premium is based on FEHB Blue Cross–Blue Shield standard national plan. Using Government Employees Health Association high national benefit plan (2006 annual premiums are $5,174 for individuals and $11,216 for families), the total non-Medicare costs would be $944 billion. Adding $61.4 billion for extra use by the Medicaid and currently uninsured populations yields $1,005.9 billion.

b. The average family size is 3.7 persons.

c. The uninsured and Medicaid populations are about a quarter of the insured population, and therefore the fraction of costs attributable to these groups is assumed to be approximately one-fourth of the $944.5 billion for the insured population, or $236 billion, augmented by 26 percent because of the higher cost per person of these populations, for a total of $297.4 billion. Adding the extra $61.4 billion in costs for this population ($297.4 billion minus $236 billion) to the $944.5 billion for the insured population results in a total of $1,005.9 billion.

d. Using estimates from 2006 according to figures cited in Catlin and others 2008.

e. Excludes payments for nursing homes.

ture on health care yet would cover everyone with essentially the same plan that covers members of Congress, even taking into account the higher use by the currently uninsured and Medicaid populations.

Much of the $1,006 billion would replace existing spending, both private and public. Moving Medicare, Medicaid, and SCHIP beneficiaries into the Guaranteed Health Care Access Plan would yield further savings. First, the need for safety net providers for the uninsured—county hospitals, community clinics, and the like—would be obviated because all Americans would have health coverage. This should reduce the health care expenditures of municipal and state governments. Second, the responsibility of state and municipal governments for funding of health care for their own employees would be eliminated, thus saving these governments even more. For instance, in 2006 almost 3 percent of Maryland's state budget went to health insurance for state workers (Office of the Governor 2005). This would be saved. Third, as new enrollment in Medicaid and SCHIP stops, and as current beneficiaries get jobs or choose to enroll in the Guaranteed Health Care Access Plan and cease to be eligible for these programs, demands on state budgets will rapidly decline. According to the National Governors Association, on average Medicaid accounted for 22 percent of state budgets, and total health care spending constituted 32 percent of state budgets.[6] Thus the combination of eliminating state responsibility for employee health insurance, phasing out Medicaid and SCHIP, and reducing support for other governmental safety net health programs would save states about 32 percent of their budgets. Although states and municipalities may choose not to reduce taxes by the full amount they save—they may instead reallocate some of the savings to other activities, such as education—their citizens should see substantial declines in state and municipal taxes along with improvements in services. The federal government would also realize substantial savings from phasing out Medicaid and SCHIP.

The total phasing out of Medicare would constitute yet another important change in taxes. With no new enrollment, the number of Medicare enrollees would decrease by about 5 or 6 percent a year because of mortality, and the program would draw to a close in a few decades. This would allow Medicare taxes—currently 2.9 percent of payroll—to be phased out. There would also be a decrease in the general federal revenue devoted to Medicare to make up for shortfalls in the trust fund. In short, the phase-out

6. National Governors Association, "Fiscal Survey of the States June 2007" (www.nasbo.org/Publications/PDFs/Fiscal%20Survey%20of%20the%20States%20June%202007.pdf).

of Medicare would rapidly result in a substantial reduction in Medicare expenditure.

How is it possible to insure all Americans for what is being paid for health care today? First, insurance underwriting, sales, and marketing costs would be significantly lower under the Guaranteed Health Care Access Plan than under the current system of employer-based insurance and self-insurance. Rather than selling to millions of individual employers—having to underwrite and market to each one—insurance companies would enter an insurance exchange that pools millions of lives and would receive risk-adjusted premiums. The resulting savings alone should be about $70 to $100 billion. In addition, employers would save the cost of administering health care benefits. Also, although the FEHB program is generous, some Americans have even more generous benefit packages. They would be entitled to fewer benefits than they currently receive through their employer-based insurance and would have to pay for any additional services. That additional cost is not included in the above figures.

Comparing the Guaranteed Health Care Access Plan with Mandates and Single-Payer Plans

Table 4-3 summarizes the principal differences between the proposed Guaranteed Health Care Access Plan and proposals for mandates and single-payer systems. Unlike mandates, universal health care vouchers would simply and efficiently achieve universal coverage without the costly administration of income-based subsidies. The poor and the sick would be implicitly subsidized by the difference between the value of the health care certificate to them and the amount of VAT they pay. Also, unlike mandates, the Guaranteed Health Care Access Plan would not prop up an inefficient and inequitable employer-based insurance system, nor would it require beneficiaries to change health plans when their income, employment, marital status, or other characteristics change. Finally, because the Guaranteed Health Care Access Plan would be universal, allowing no denial of coverage, it would not be subject to the adverse selection problem in which a disproportionate share of higher users of care are drawn into the system while individuals or employers with better insurance risks make other arrangements. Individual or employer mandates that use voluntary insurance exchanges by themselves remain subject to this serious problem.

One very important difference between the Guaranteed Health Care Access Plan and single-payer systems currently proposed is that the latter

Table 4-3. Comparison of the Proposed Guaranteed Health Care Access Plan with Other Proposals

Criterion	Guaranteed Health Care Access Plan	Individual and/or employer mandates	Single-payer plans
Universal coverage	True universal coverage of all Americans.	Falls short of universal coverage. Requires everyone to have insurance coverage through an employer, government, or self-purchase, but some people will evade mandates and others will be exempted because coverage is unaffordable.	True universal coverage of all Americans.
Choice	Every American has a choice of health plan, hospital, and physicians.	Many people insured through their employer continue to have no choice of health plan. People insured through Medicaid still have very limited choice.	Every American has a choice of hospital and physicians but is enrolled in a single nationwide plan.
Role of employers	Employers are taken completely out of the health care system. Consequently, wages increase and strikes over health insurance disappear. Neither workers nor employers any longer make job decisions based on health insurance considerations.	Employers remain involved in health care as they are now. Employers who drop insurance coverage for their workers may pay a penalty.	Employers are taken completely out of the health care system.
Cost control	Controls costs through several mechanisms: a dedicated tax that links spending on health care to willingness to pay taxes, competition between health plans, greater cost consciousness on the part of individuals buying additional services, systematic technology assessment that eliminates practices of marginal or no value, and incentives that shift research and development by drug and medical device companies toward more cost-effective interventions.	No cost control mechanism.	Controls costs through negotiation of fees, prices, and budgets with physicians, hospitals, drug companies, and other providers, and through restrictions on the supply of medical technologies.

Administrative efficiency	Administrative costs are about 10 percent of total health care spending. Administrative savings are achieved by reducing insurance underwriting, sales, and marketing, and through administration cuts by employers. The elimination of the administrative burden of Medicaid and of the income-linked determination of subsidies would also create administrative efficiencies.	Administrative costs exceed 15 or 20 percent, with no administrative savings. The need to determine incomes and the level of subsidies provided to individuals to buy health insurance would increase costs.	Administrative costs of about 3 to 4 percent. Administrative savings are achieved by removing employers as well as all insurance companies and for-profit providers from the health care system.
Technology and outcomes assessment	Creates an Institute for Technology and Outcomes Assessment to evaluate the effectiveness and cost of drugs, devices, and new technologies and to evaluate patient outcomes and the quality performance of health plans and insurance companies.	No systematic effort to assess technology or outcomes.	No systematic effort to assess technology or outcomes.
Delivery system	Provides strong incentives, through financing and data collection by the regional health boards, for health plans to integrate care across hospitals, physicians, and other providers.	Same health care delivery system as at present. No financial or other incentive to create accountable health plans or integrate care.	Same health care delivery system as at present. No financial or other incentive to create accountable health plans or integrate care.

promise an open-ended entitlement that is often not tied directly to adequate funding. In the Guaranteed Health Care Access Plan, by contrast, expenditure and revenue are explicitly connected through the dedicated tax. Also, single-payer systems generally provide only a monetary promise; they do not guarantee access to care. Medicaid beneficiaries and increasingly Medicare beneficiaries have difficulty finding a physician to accept them as patients because of low fees paid by the government. In the Guaranteed Health Care Access Plan, everyone would be enrolled in a plan that is held responsible for providing care to its enrollees.

Finally, a crucial difference between the Guaranteed Health Care Access Plan and the other two models is that neither of the other two models makes a significant effort to improve efficiency in the organization and delivery of care. The proposed Guaranteed Health Care Access Plan, by contrast, would make plans accountable for quality and service by allowing only qualified plans to enroll patients. Paying a risk-adjusted fee per enrollee (that is, capitation) creates a strong financial incentive for insurance companies to be efficient in care delivery. In short, the projected universal voucher system would be more than just a funding mechanism. It would create a positive dynamic that moves the entire system toward more efficient use of resources and higher-quality care.

What Would the Health Care Experience Be Like under the Guaranteed Health Care Access Plan?

Initially, all Americans not in Medicare, Medicaid, or SCHIP would be notified by their regional health board that they can now choose their health plan or health insurance company through the insurance exchange. Through mailings, the Internet, and other mechanisms, potential enrollees would be informed about the different plans available in their geographic area. Charts would identify the similarities and differences in the various plans: what local hospitals each plan uses, the physicians participating in the plan, the copayments required, and other relevant information. In addition, potential enrollees would have data on the patient outcomes in each health plan to assess the comparative quality of care provided. Americans would also be instructed on how to enroll. People with coverage today would be able to keep their current doctor, and many aspects of their plan would remain the same.

As stated above, Medicare, Medicaid, SCHIP, and other government health programs would initially remain in place, but participants in these programs would be notified that they could now switch to the Guaranteed

Health Care Access Plan. Those who prefer not to switch would just stay in their current program.

For most Americans, enrollment in a health plan or insurance company under the Guaranteed Health Care Access Plan would feel much like what they currently experience through their employer-based coverage, with five important differences. First, they would have a wider choice of health plans. Today most Americans who are covered by their employer have no choice of health plan (Kaiser Family Foundation 2006). They are told by their employer who will provide their coverage and what services will be covered. Those currently uninsured and the self-insured would experience a new freedom to choose a health plan.

Second, Americans would no longer have to be screened to determine their premiums or to determine what will be excluded from coverage for the first year. No health plan or insurance company would be allowed to subject Americans to pretesting or to deny coverage on the basis of preexisting conditions. No one could be denied enrollment or renewal of coverage for any reason. Instead of health plans choosing their enrollees, as is effectively the case today, enrollees would be allowed to choose their health plan.

Third, in choosing a health plan or insurance company, Americans would have reliable data comparing the quality of the various alternatives. Through the regional health boards, the health plans and insurance companies would have to regularly report results for quality indicators defined by the National Health Board. These indicators might include rates of hospitalization for diabetic patients, thirty-day mortality rates for patients with heart attacks, and rates of the use of appropriate chemotherapies for different cancers. This would provide Americans with reliable quality data they do not have now to make informed decisions.

Fourth, enrollees would pay nothing directly for the set of standard health benefits. The health care certificate would cover the full cost of the standard benefits plan. There would be no premiums deducted from paychecks or paid for out of pocket. There would be no deductibles, and many people would find their copayments to be less than what they are currently paying.

Fifth, enrollees could decide whether they want to buy additional services or insurance coverage, and how much they are willing to pay for them.

Workers who currently receive health coverage through their employer—whether they work in a factory, an office, or a government agency—would see more money in their paycheck as employers compete for their labor by offering higher wages instead of health benefits (Emanuel and Fuchs 2008; Gruber 2000). Fringe benefits such as health coverage are, after all, just another form of compensation (Gruber 2000). When employers stop offering health insurance, the money that before went into health insurance premiums would be offered instead to workers as higher salaries to induce them to stay with the company. How much would workers' pay rise? It would primarily depend on how much of current workers' compensation is in the form of health insurance.

Conversely, Americans would for the first time pay a VAT. Over time, as Medicare and Medicaid are phased out and their beneficiaries are enrolled in the voucher system, it would increase from the initial 10 to 12 percent to approximately 15 percent. The new tax would be offset by the higher wages mentioned above and by reductions in other taxes. Each year the federal government would pay less and less for Medicare, Medicaid, SCHIP, and other programs, reducing the strain on federal finances and taxes. Similarly, states would pay less and less for Medicaid, SCHIP, and other need-based programs, for state workers' health insurance, and for safety net providers—including county hospitals, community health clinics, and other programs. Eventually, when the Guaranteed Health Care Access Plan is fully implemented, these programs could be eliminated or integrated into the health system. Overall, as calculated above, elimination of state expenditures devoted to health care programs would reduce total state expenditures by a substantial 32 percent.

People with diabetes, emphysema, heart failure, and other chronic conditions would probably experience much better coordination of care: more home visits from nurses to be sure they are taking their medicine and following the treatment plan, and more telephone calls and other reminders to check on their diet and their use of medications and vaccines. They also would probably observe a greater effort to involve them in exercise, smoking cessation programs, and other preventive activities. Capitation payment to the health plans as well as the need to report quality indicators would lead them to emphasize keeping enrollees well.

Potential Concerns about the Guaranteed Health Care Access Plan

Three main obstacles stand in the way of enacting the Guaranteed Health Care Access Plan. First is the perception on the part of many that a VAT would be regressive and would hurt the poor. Although this contention is widely repeated, it is simplistic at best. The fairness of any tax proposal cannot be properly evaluated by considering only the tax. The United States currently has a more progressive tax system—measured by reductions in the Gini coefficient—than Norway or Sweden.[7] This means that taxes alone do not determine overall progressivity of government spending. The benefits that the tax would pay for must also be considered—as well as the costs and benefits of alternative policies or of doing nothing. The current financing of the health care system is structured largely around the generous tax benefits, worth over $200 billion in 2007, given to employer-based insurance. The system is heavily biased toward the rich and against the less well off.[8] Not only do the rich receive a bigger tax break, but the working poor often pay Medicare and other taxes yet receive no health coverage in return. Under the Guaranteed Health Care Access Plan, everyone would pay the VAT in proportion to their consumption.

The essential point, however, is that less-well-off Americans—as well as all those who are sick and therefore need more health care services—would generally receive much more in benefits than they would pay in taxes. Health coverage for a family in 2008 costs over $12,000 a year. The poor, the near poor, and many other people earning less than the median income would not pay anywhere near that much in value-added taxes. Consequently, the value of the health coverage they receive would greatly exceed what they pay in tax for that coverage. That is the hallmark of progressivity—and that, not progressivity of taxes alone, is how other countries really achieve reductions in income inequality.

A second obstacle is the danger that insurance companies and health plan sponsors might find ways to cherry-pick (or "lemon drop") prospective customers in a system that allows all Americans to choose among competing private health plans and insurance companies. It could be profitable for a health plan or insurance company to avoid sick patients and attract young, healthy ones. Sick patients might be discouraged from signing up, for example, if a hospital network failed to include a cancer center, offered only second-rate mental health services, or did not contract with the best diabetes doctors.

Fortunately, there are ways of preventing this outcome. One important countermeasure is the requirement for guarantee issue, renewability, and the prevention of exempting preexisting conditions. But the real key to prevent adverse selection is risk adjustment. The regional health boards would pay health plans more per patient if they enroll older, sicker patients on

7. Lane Kenworthy, "Taxes and Inequality: Lessons from Abroad" (lanekenworthy.net/2008/02/10/taxes-and-inequality-lessons-from-abroad/)

8. John Sheils and Randall Haught, "The Cost of Tax-Exempt Health Benefits in 2004," *Health Affairs,* web exclusive, February 15, 2004 (content.healthaffairs.org/cgi/reprint/hlthaff.w4.106v1.pdf).

average, and less if they enroll young, healthy people. Some health care systems in the United States and health authorities in some other countries, such as the Netherlands and Israel, already have relevant experience with what risk adjustment does and does not work. This experience could be applied to the Guaranteed Health Care Access Plan. Admittedly, risk adjustment is still an imperfect science. The National Health Board would need to conduct research into improving adjustment methods. In the meantime, however, there could be some form of reinsurance. For instance, regional health boards could provide "stop-loss" coverage, so that any plan that spends more than $100,000 on a single patient is not held liable for the full cost; the regional health board would pick up the excess. But however it is accomplished, some form of risk adjustment is critical to a stable, efficient, and fair program, and to ensuring that the system focuses resources on providing the best health care for people who are sick, not on coddling the worried well.

The final hurdle that the Guaranteed Health Care Access Plan must overcome is political. This plan constitutes a comprehensive reform of the U.S. health care system. It would mean change in the way health care insurance is financed, in the role of employers, in the way the system is administered, in the way Americans enroll, in the way the system delivers care, and in the way technology is developed and evaluated. Such far-reaching change is sure to create uncertainty, and uncertainty makes people cautious. Overcoming such inertia and innate risk aversion is a challenge facing any serious health care reform. What ultimately emerges will depend on a balance of factors: how bad the current system has become, how willing people are to try something new, and how much they can be convinced that what is being proposed has a good chance of being better.

Advantages of the Guaranteed Health Care Access Plan

Compared with the current health care system, the Guaranteed Health Care Access Plan offers advantages in almost every area: coverage and choice, administrative efficiency, cost control, quality, and impact on the economy (Emanuel 2008).

COVERAGE AND CHOICE. With no restrictions or enrollment requirements, guaranteed issue and renewability, and no exclusions for preexisting health conditions, the Guaranteed Health Care Access Plan would guarantee that every American has health coverage—not 95 or 97 or even 99 percent of Americans, but 100 percent. Even those who fail to sign up for a health plan would be assigned a plan and would be covered. There would be no gaps.

Americans would enjoy both continuity of coverage and choice. As long as they wanted to stay in a health plan or with a particular physician, they could do so. They could not be denied coverage or denied renewal of their plan. Their employer could not switch plans or force them to change physicians or hospitals. Each individual would decide whether and when to switch health plans, physicians, or hospitals and whether or not to buy additional services beyond those in the standard health benefit. Each household would be allowed to weigh whether a wider choice of physicians and hospitals or coverage for complementary medicine is worth the money that could otherwise be spent on, say, sending their children to a private college or buying a new car.

ADMINISTRATIVE EFFICIENCY. Eliminating the employer from health coverage and removing the burden of Medicaid administration on states would create significant administrative savings and efficiencies, as described above. Putting all Americans—initially everyone except those who choose to remain in Medicare, Medicaid, SCHIP, or another government program—into the insurance exchange would save tens of billions of dollars that are now spent on insurance underwriting, sales, and marketing. Since the Guaranteed Health Care Access Plan would require no determination of eligibility for participation or for subsidies based on income, its adoption would produce additional billions in administrative savings. Employers also would save billions because they would no longer need such large human resources departments to manage health benefits and track health contributions, nor would they need to hire consultants to evaluate various insurance options. Once phase-in is complete, states would no longer have to administer Medicaid, and providers would no longer have to bill Medicaid, producing still more efficiency.

The Guaranteed Health Care Access Plan would lead to a reduction in the number of health plans and insurance companies. There are more than 1,000 such companies that operate today; these would probably consolidate to fewer than 100 or so companies nationwide, with many fewer in any one city or region. This would lead to significant savings in billing costs at hospitals and physicians' offices. As Medicare, Medicaid, SCHIP, and other government programs are phased out, hospitals, physicians' offices, home health agencies, and others would realize additional administrative savings because they would be dealing with even fewer billing systems.

The administrative costs of the Guaranteed Health Care Access Plan would not be as low as those of a single-payer system. Expenditures for the proposed Institute for Technology and Outcomes Assessment (an estimated

0.5 percent of costs) and for the Centers for Patient Safety and Dispute Resolution (2.5 percent), as well as for the national and regional health boards, would probably amount to 10 percent of the system's total cost. Even with these costs, however, more than $100 billion in administrative savings would be realized each year. Furthermore, the information generated by some of the administrative expenditures, such as the quality of care provided by the various health plans and insurance companies, would be invaluable in improving quality and enhancing the value of health expenditures. This would be administrative cost *with* benefits—a benefit the current system cannot realize.

COST CONTROL. Another major advantage of the Guaranteed Health Care Access Plan would be effective cost control, which would ensure the financial sustainability of the entire health care system. This would be achieved without price controls on fees for physicians and hospitals or the centralized management of local spending constitutive of current single-payer proposals. There would be five separate cost control levers. First, and most effectively, the yield from the VAT would determine how much could be spent on the overall health care system. This would provide a hard budget constraint on cost increases. Of course, revenue collected by the VAT would rise as the economy grows; but if the public wanted health care spending to grow even more rapidly because it wanted additional services, it would have to persuade Congress to increase the tax rate. Americans' aversion to tax increases should thus hold health care costs down, but the system would allow Congress to enact increases when the public deems the added expenditure as value for money.

Second, competition among health plans would restrain costs. Currently, competition among health plans is perverse. Plans do not compete to offer a package of services for a fixed price. Instead, all too frequently they compete to avoid sick patients. Under the Guaranteed Health Care Access Plan, because health plans and insurance companies would have the same risk-adjusted fixed payment per enrollee for a standard set of benefits, with no opportunity to charge enrollees more for those benefits, they would have to compete for enrollees. They would therefore have a strong financial incentive to be efficient. The likely result would be innovations in the management of chronic illnesses, where 70 percent of health care spending occurs (Agency for Healthcare Research 2002). Because hospitalization is so expensive, health plans would probably find ways to keep patients with chronic conditions healthier and out of the hospital. Similarly, they would have a strong incentive to eliminate duplicate testing and expensive medicine that adds little or no benefit.

Third, those Americans who want additional services would have to pay for them with after-tax dollars. They would therefore have an incentive to spend judiciously to receive value for their money.

Fourth, the independent Institute for Technology and Outcomes Assessment would evaluate the effectiveness, cost, and value of new technologies and new applications of existing technologies. Data developed by the institute would ensure that any new procedures added to coverage under the standard benefit package would be cost effective; the data would also provide vital information for health plans and insurance companies as they design more efficient and effective care. Data from the institute would ensure that any cost cutting that harms patients would be detected. Health plans could also cover only cost-effective, proven care without fear of litigation since the Centers for Patient Safety and Dispute Resolution, which would adjudicate claims of medical error, would not view use of evaluations by the institute as a medical error. This would provide a safe harbor for actual implementation of cost-effective care by health plans.

Finally, the institute's reports would send a signal to drug and medical device companies to focus their research and development on cost-effective interventions. Right now, the new interventions that these companies develop are typically expected to hit the market in ten years. Companies thus face uncertainty about what interventions will be covered by health insurers ten years hence, and at what price. They therefore try to recoup their costs as fast as possible through high prices. The institute would provide more reliable and predictable information on future coverage decisions, emphasizing that cost-effective interventions—those that really improve survival or quality of life, or that save money without reducing the quality of care—will be covered. This would lead to a shift in research priorities and hold down costs in the future.

No single cost control mechanism is likely to be effective in restraining the rise in health care expenditure, but these five different mechanisms all pulling in the same direction should together make a difference.

IMPROVED QUALITY. The Guaranteed Health Care Access Plan would also improve quality and patient safety, especially through innovation in health care delivery. Today we know two things about quality: that the current system does not consistently deliver high-quality care and that health plans and current practitioners do not know the best way to deliver high-quality care. Innovation in health care delivery is desperately needed.

Hospitals and health professionals today have few financial or other incentives to implement patient safety measures. The Guaranteed Health

Care Access Plan would provide strong incentives for health plans and insurance companies to develop infrastructure that improves quality. Monitoring of outcomes by the Institute for Technology and Outcomes Assessment and monitoring of health plan performance by the National Health Board would provide significant incentives for health plans to invest in information technologies, including computer order entry systems for physicians, electronic medical records, and other ways to share data. The regional Centers for Patient Safety and Dispute Resolution would develop and finance interventions to improve patient safety.

The Guaranteed Health Care Access Plan would end the malpractice nightmare in which thousands of patients who are injured are never compensated while a few patients reap outsized rewards, and in which doctors practice defensive medicine while paying large malpractice premiums. To cut through this morass, the Guaranteed Health Care Access Plan's Centers for Patient Safety and Dispute Resolution would adjudicate all patient claims of injury and compensate quickly and fairly those who have actually suffered harm. The money would come not from malpractice premiums but from the VAT. This would largely free physicians from the malpractice burden, but in exchange they would have to agree that the bad physicians who cause a disproportionate amount of malpractice injury will be drummed out of the profession.

In short, unlike individual mandates or single-payer plans, the universal voucher proposal deals with both malpractice and patient safety more broadly. Many interventions that would improve patient safety have not been implemented, despite substantial evidence that they really reduce infections, reduce complications, and save money and lives. There are many reasons for this inaction, but surely one of them is that no organization exists today with the muscle and money to push for change. The Guaranteed Health Care Access Plan would provide both the impetus and the money to develop interventions and implement them.

ECONOMIC IMPROVEMENT. The Guaranteed Health Care Access Plan would help the economy. Most obviously, it would relieve businesses of the burden of financing and administering their employees' health insurance, thus making them more efficient and competitive. Employers would also be relieved of obligations for their retirees' health coverage, and they could reduce spending on human resources departments and consultants, freeing resources to invest in their core business. They would no longer have to cope with the unpredictability of future health care cost increases, and they could once again base hiring decisions on demand for their output and on worker productivity, not on the basis of future health care costs. This should boost employment.

The Guaranteed Health Care Access Plan would also be a huge benefit for workers. Their health care coverage would be guaranteed, not tied to their job and possibly lost if they are laid off. Strikes over health benefits would disappear. The phenomenon of job lock, in which workers stay in jobs where they are no longer happy or productive so as not to lose their health insurance coverage, would vanish. Although they would pay a new tax, the VAT, workers would at the same time see their Medicare taxes, federal income taxes, and state taxes decline, and they would likely receive pay increases in lieu of the health insurance benefits they formerly received. Over time, with effective cost control, pay increases would once again reflect increases in productivity and not be held down by increases in health care premiums.

OTHER ADVANTAGES. Two of the biggest advantages of the Guaranteed Health Care Access Plan are implicit rather than explicit. The first is that the plan is comparatively simple. The second is that it coheres with American values.

Nothing that changes the way $1 out of every $6 is raised and spent in the U.S. economy is going to be very simple, but the Guaranteed Health Care Access Plan has relatively few moving parts—fewer than the current complex health system. It envisages one standard benefits plan for all Americans. Using implicit subsidies through taxes, it involves no income-linked subsidies and thus entails none of the complex administration that such subsidies require. It relies on just one funding source, the VAT, rather than on many different streams—employer contributions, worker premiums, out-of-pocket costs, Medicare taxes, and other state and federal taxes. Each region of the country would have just one insurance exchange. The number of health plans and insurance companies nationwide would be substantially reduced. Employers would be freed of responsibility for financing health care. Administration of the system would be handled by one national board and twelve regional health boards. No other health care proposal that seeks significant improvement is as simple. Such simplicity makes incentives clearer and more effective instead of confusing and counterproductive.

The Guaranteed Health Care Access Plan's biggest advantage, however, may be the way it reflects core American values: equality of opportunity and individual freedom. The United States is different from many other Western countries that emphasize an egalitarian ethos. The Guaranteed

Health Care Access Plan would promote equality of opportunity: its standard benefits would be provided to everyone, funded by a tax that everyone pays and cannot evade. At the same time, it would let individual freedom flourish: it would use market mechanisms—competition—to foster quality and efficiency in health plans and in hospital and physician delivery of services. It would give people a choice of health plans, physicians, and hospitals operating in the private sector, and the option to spend their own money to buy more coverage for amenities and a wider range of services. This balance of equality of opportunity with market mechanisms and individual freedom is quintessentially American.

If Americans want a health care financing system that can achieve universal coverage, with multiple cost control mechanisms and incentives to improve quality, and one that can do so in a sustainable way, the Guaranteed Health Care Access Plan is the best option.

References

Agency for Healthcare Research and Quality. 2002. "Health Care Costs." Fact sheet. U.S. Department of Health and Human Services.

Boards of Trustees. 2007. *2007 Annual Report of the Boards of Trustees, Federal Hospital Insurance and Federal Supplementary Medical Insurance Trust Funds.*

Butler, Stuart M. 2001. "Reforming the Tax Treatment of Health Care to Achieve Universal Coverage." In *Covering America: Real Remedies for the Uninsured*, edited by Eliot K. Wicks, pp. 23–42. Washington: Economic and Social Research Institute.

Catlin, Aaron, and others. 2008. "National Health Spending in 2006: A Year of Change for Prescription Drugs." *Health Affairs* 27, no. 1:14–29.

Congressional Budget Office. 2004. "Limiting Tort Liability for Medical Malpractice." Economic and Budget Issue Brief (January).

Emanuel, Ezekiel. 2008. *Healthcare, Guaranteed: A Simple, Secure Solution for America.* New York: PublicAffairs.

Emanuel, Ezekiel, and Victor Fuchs. 2005. "Health Care Vouchers: A Proposal for Universal Coverage." *New England Journal of Medicine* 352, no. 12: 1255–60.

———. 2008. "Who Really Pays for Health Care? The Myth of 'Shared Responsibility.'" *Journal of the American Medical Association* 299, no. 9:1057–59.

Enthoven, Alain, and Richard Kronick. 1989. "A Consumer-Choice Health Plan for the 1990s: Universal Health Insurance in a System Designed to Promote Quality and Economy." *New England Journal of Medicine* 320, no. 2: 29–37, 94–101.

Fuchs, Victor, and Ezekiel Emanuel. 2005. "Health Care Reform: Why? What? When?" *Health Affairs* 24, no. 6: 1399–414.

Gruber, Jonathan. 2000. "Health Insurance and the Labor Market." In *Handbook of Health Economics,* vol. 1A, edited by Joseph P. Newhouse and Anthony J. Culyer, pp. 645–706. Amsterdam: North Holland.

———. 2006. "The Massachusetts Health Care Revolution: A Local Start for Universal Access." *Hastings Center Report* 36, no. 5: 14–19.

Holahan, John, Randall Bovbjerg, and Jack Hadley. 2006. "Caring for the Uninsured in Massachusetts: What Does It Cost, Who Pays, and What Would Full Coverage Add to Medical Spending." Research report. Washington: Urban Institute.

Kaiser Family Foundation and Health Research and Educational Trust. 2006. *Employer Health Benefits: 2006 Annual Survey.* Menlo Park, Calif., and Chicago.

Linda T. Kohn, Janet M. Corrigan, and Molla S. Donaldson, eds. 2000. *To Err Is Human: Building a Safer Health System. Committee on Quality of Health Care in America.* Washington: National Academies Press.

Mangione-Smith, Rita, and others. 2007. "The Quality of Ambulatory Care Delivered to Children in the United States." *New England Journal of Medicine* 357, no. 15: 1515–23.

McGlynn, Elizabeth, and others. 2003. "The Quality of Health Care Delivered to Adults in the United States." *New England Journal of Medicine* 348, no. 26: 2635–45.

Office of the Governor. 2005. *The 5 Pillars of the Ehrlich-Steele Administration.* Annapolis, Md.

Palmisano, Donald J., David W. Emmons, and Gregory D. Wozniak. 2004. "Expanding Insurance Coverage through Tax Credits, Consumer Choice, and Market Enhancements: The American Medical Association Proposal for Insurance Reform." *Journal of the American Medical Association* 291, no. 18: 2237–42.

Pauly, Mark V. 2001. "An Adaptive Credit Plan for Covering the Uninsured." In *Covering America: Real Remedies for the Uninsured,* edited by Eliot K. Wicks, pp. 137–52. Washington: Economic and Social Research Institute.

Physicians' Working Group. 2003. "Proposal of the Physicians' Working Group for Single-Payer National Health Insurance." *Journal of the American Medical Association* 290, no. 6: 798–805.

Wachter, Robert M., and Kaveh G. Shojania. 2004. *Internal Bleeding: The Truth behind America's Terrifying Epidemic of Medical Mistakes.* New York: Rugged Land Press.

Taking Massachusetts National

Incremental Universalism for the United States

5

JONATHAN GRUBER

The history of health care reform in the United States is littered with failed attempts at universal health care coverage. The most recent was the Clinton Health Security Act of 1993–94, which proposed an ambitious overhaul of the U.S. health care system; it was defeated soundly in Congress. There has been no serious national attempt at universal coverage since that time. For example, in 2004, Democratic presidential candidate John F. Kerry focused much more on lowering health insurance premiums than he did on broad expansions of coverage.

All of this has changed recently, but this time the states are taking the lead. Most notable has been the health reform plan enacted by Massachusetts in April 2006. This sweeping bill reformed insurance markets, subsidized insurance coverage for a large swath of the population, introduced a new purchasing mechanism (the Health Connector, or the "Connector"), and mandated insurance coverage for almost all citizens. The success to date of the effort in Massachusetts has led to similar proposals in a number of states, most notably the proposal in California by Governor Arnold

Jonathan Gruber is professor of public finance at the Massachusetts Institute of Technology and is an economist with the National Bureau of Economic Research. This paper was prepared for The Hamilton Project Conference "Health Care Reconsidered: Options for Change, Part Two: Who's Got the Cure? Four Options for Achieving Universal Coverage," July 17, 2007.

Schwarzenegger. The Massachusetts bill, perhaps, has also been the motivation in 2008 for similar proposals from the leading Democratic presidential candidates.

This chapter discusses a plan for taking the Massachusetts model to a national scale. I begin by discussing the structure of the Massachusetts reform, highlighting the major issues that were faced in the first year of implementing this reform and how I would resolve these issues in a national plan. I then provide estimates of the cost, coverage, and distributional implications of such a reform, using a microsimulation model developed to assess the cost and coverage impacts of reform proposals.

Next, I turn to the important issue of financing. I estimate that replicating this plan at the national level would cost about $130 billion a year in 2007 dollars. There is a natural source of financing that can more than cover this total: the tax subsidy to employer-provided health insurance. In the final section of the paper, I discuss the important distributional implications of financing universal coverage using this revenue source.

Universal Coverage: What Are the Issues?

Who Are the Uninsured?

There are currently 47 million uninsured individuals in the United States. Who are they? According to data from the Current Population Survey, the uninsured have lower-than-average incomes: nearly two-thirds of the uninsured are in families with incomes below double the poverty line.[1] Not all the uninsured, however, are low income. Twenty-eight percent of the uninsured are in families with incomes above $50,000 a year. Sixty-three percent of the uninsured are in families where the family head is a full-time, full-year worker but is either not offered health insurance or does not enroll to cover him- or herself or family members. Several million of the uninsured are undocumented immigrants, who are generally not eligible for public programs. Thus the modal uninsured person is a member of the *working-poor class:* below median income but not among the poorest in the nation (Employee Benefit Research Institute 2007).

Significantly more than 47 million people lack health insurance at some point during any given year. Although the Current Population Survey data underlying the statistics in the previous paragraph are based on a question asking whether people were uninsured during the entire previous year,

1. U.S. Census Bureau, "Current Population Survey" (www.census.gov/cps/). The U.S. "poverty threshold" in 2008 for a family of four is $20,650.

most analysts suspect that respondents are replying about current insurance status. For example, the Congressional Budget Office (CBO) finds that other surveys that ask about uninsurance at a particular point in the year provide estimates very similar to the Current Population Survey (CBO 2003). The CBO finds that estimates of uninsurance over an *entire* calendar year are only about one-half to two-thirds as large as point-in-time estimates, however, and that estimates of the number of individuals uninsured *at any point* in the last year are about 40–50 percent higher than point-in-time estimates. These findings highlight the dynamic nature of uninsurance.

Why Universal Coverage?

Does the simple fact that 18 percent of the nonelderly population lacks health insurance necessarily make that a major social policy problem? Many more than 18 percent of the population do not own their own homes or are obese. So why should we care about uninsurance in the United States?

First, the classic argument for increasing insurance coverage is based on the externalities associated with underinsurance. For example, there are physical externalities associated with communicable diseases: uninsured people are less likely to receive vaccinations and to care of communicable diseases. Since such a small share of medical expenditures is related to communicable disease, however, this is not a major rationale for universal health insurance (as opposed to universal vaccination). There is also a financial externality imposed by the uninsured on the insured through uncompensated care. When the uninsured do not pay their medical bills, their costs are passed on to other users of the medical system. Such uncompensated care amounts to only $30 billion each year, a small amount relative to the $2 trillion health economy.

Second, increasing coverage could eliminate inefficiencies associated with uninsurance. One such concern is labor market distortion caused by employer-based coverage. It is possible that many individuals are afraid of losing their health insurance coverage, which makes them unwilling to search for or to move to jobs where they would be more productive. This reluctance to change can lead to a mismatch between workers and jobs that can lower overall U.S. productivity. This situation is referred to as *job lock:* the unwillingness of an individual to move to a better job for fear of losing health insurance.[2] Empirical studies, reviewed in Gruber and

---

2. See Gruber (2001) for a discussion of the theory of job lock.

Madrian (2004), confirm that mobility from job to job is reduced by job lock; Madrian (1994) estimates that job lock may reduce mobility by as much as 25 percent. At the same time, the fact that mobility is reduced does not necessarily have major welfare implications, an issue that has received relatively little attention. Gruber and Madrian (2004) offer some back-of-the-envelope calculations that suggest that the welfare cost is unlikely to be large—only about $15 billion to $30 billion. These are very rough calculations, though, and this is an area of considerable uncertainty.

A third economic argument in favor of government intervention for universal insurance is the notion that asymmetric information can cause adverse selection, leading to market failure. In the case of health insurance—for example, if the potential insured person knows more about her preexisting conditions than she reveals—insurance companies might offer incomplete insurance in order to deter high-risk types. This situation might even lead to a "death spiral" of rising premiums and an increasingly risky pool of insured persons that eventually leads to the collapse of the market. In these circumstances, government intervention through a mandate or regulation can improve welfare.

A fourth concern with the uninsured is the issue of affordability. As discussed below, health insurance is very expensive, and many individuals who might rationally demand health insurance cannot afford it at current prices. This leads to an argument for covering the uninsured as a form of redistribution.

The final motivation for caring about the uninsured is what economists would call *paternalism:* the concern that individuals without health insurance may be harming themselves by not buying insurance. There is a clear belief among the public and policymakers that being uninsured is bad for your health. An Institute of Medicine (IOM) study reviewed hundreds of studies documenting the health problems associated with uninsurance (IOM 2001). That study estimates that uninsured individuals use only half as much medical care as the insured use and have a mortality risk that is 25 percent higher, with more than 18,000 people dying each year because of lack of insurance (IOM 2001). While the studies reviewed by the IOM were mostly observational analyses documenting a correlation between a lack of health insurance and poor health, several other studies have used careful empirical methods to document more carefully a causal impact of health insurance on health (Currie and Gruber 1996a, 1996b; Hanratty 1996; Lurie and others 1984).

What Are the Issues?

Any approach to universal insurance coverage in the United States must address three critical issues: pooling, affordability, and mandates.

POOLING. The efficient provision of insurance requires large pools of participants that are created independent of health status (that is, health status that the insurer does not or cannot observe). Absent such pools, insurers will be reluctant to offer insurance, or will do so only with incomplete coverage or at very high prices, for fear of adverse selection and high-cost exposure. The majority of Americans can access insurance through such pools, either through large firms or through publicly provided insurance. Most of the uninsured, however, do not have access to any such pooling mechanism. For example, most uninsured persons do not work for an employer that offers insurance. Solving the problem of the uninsured requires developing some new pooling mechanism, either through government insurance or through private insurance–purchasing arrangements such as the Federal Employees Health Benefits Plan. The success of attempts to create a new pool will depend on scale: existing state-level attempts to create pools for small businesses have generally failed because they did not attract a sufficient number of enrollees to deal with concerns about adverse selection and to spread administrative costs.

AFFORDABILITY. Health insurance is expensive. The average cost to a family for health insurance offered through large firms in Massachusetts is about $12,000 a year. It is even higher for those who work for small firms, and higher still for those who are in the nongroup market. For a family of four with combined income of $40,000 (about 200 percent of the poverty line), for example, family coverage would cost about one-third of family income, a huge share of income to devote solely to health care. What is an "affordable" level of health insurance spending? There is no correct answer for all, but these high costs highlight the fact that it is impossible for the government to reduce substantially the number of uninsured individuals without providing large subsidies to low-income groups to cover the costs of insurance.

MANDATES. Even large subsidies for health insurance coverage will not be sufficient to end the problem of uninsurance. As noted above, more than one-third of the uninsured are eligible for either free public insurance or highly subsidized employer-provided insurance yet do not take it up. To come close to full insurance in the United States would require an individual mandate: a requirement on individuals to obtain some type of insurance coverage. This mandate would be similar to automobile insurance in most states, where individuals are required to have insurance if they own a car. Some have argued that a mandate would be hard to enforce, but there is considerable evidence that mandates can be enforced. The Netherlands and Switzerland both have compliance rates of 98 to 99 percent with their health insurance mandates. The compliance rate for auto insurance in U.S. states with high levels of information sharing is about 98 percent (Nichols, Gruber, and Pauly 2007). In addition to addressing the externality, adverse selection, and paternalism arguments set out above, another justification for mandates is that more effective risk pooling would be accomplished by the implied cross-subsidy of the sick by the healthy.

Past (Polarized) Debates

Within the framework of these three issues, we can consider the alternative approaches to universal coverage favored by the left and the right of the political spectrum.

THE LEFT. The solution favored by many on the left is to move to a single-payer system. Such a system would have a clear advantage through savings in administrative costs. Administrative costs in private insurance average about 12 percent of premiums, whereas administrative costs in the Canadian National Health Insurance program are 1.3 percent (Woolhandler, Campbell, and Himmelstein 2003). There would also be additional savings to providers from dealing with one national insurer rather than with multiple private insurers.

At the same time, there may be disadvantages from having the government set a national benefits package. The limitations of policymakers with incomplete knowledge attempting to tailor benefit packages to individual preferences in the face of rapidly changing technology could be compounded by the politicization of the benefits package selection, potentially resulting in a package that is wrong for most Americans. A lack of innovation in insurance provision could also result in missed opportunities for learning which approaches are best for benefits coverage and provider reimbursement. For example, some of the 10.7 percent differential in administrative costs between Canada and the United States is money spent on care management, which may be a cost-effective expenditure. Unfortunately, we have little hard data on the allocation. More generally, dynamic solutions to control costs may be more likely to arise from a competitive environment than from a monopoly environment. For example, most of the private firms offering prescription drug coverage through Medicare do not use the government template for their plan but instead have adopted innovative ideas such as tiered drug pricing for generics and name-brand drugs. Although it is too early for a full welfare evaluation of these innovations, they appear (at least initially) to be effective in controlling costs while maintaining quality.

Beyond the pros and cons on policy grounds, national health insurance also has serious political problems. First, the majority of Americans, particularly those working for large firms with a choice of plans, are content with their private health insurance. It would be a difficult political sell to convince those Americans that they have to give up their insurance plan choices so that a minority of Americans can gain coverage.[3] Second, the private health insurance industry in the United States is a massive entity with more than $500 billion in claims paid annually. It is impossible to conceive of a state of the world in which an industry of that size could be legislated out of business. It seems unlikely that any health insurance reform in the United States in the near future will not incorporate private health insurance.

THE RIGHT. For many on the right, the problem of uninsurance is addressed best through expanding affordability of private health insurance. For example, individuals could be given tax credits to purchase health insurance from private vendors. Modest versions of this approach were a staple of the Bush administration budget proposals in every year from 2001 through 2006.

Such an approach has the advantage of addressing directly the affordability concern noted above while maintaining the private health insurance market. However, this approach explicitly does not deal with either of the other two issues that must be addressed to move to universal coverage. Currently, individuals who do not have access to either large employer pools or public insurance, particularly those without any employer insurance offering, face an insurance market that features high and variable premiums, and insurance coverage that is often incomplete. Providing individuals with more resources without giving them a place to take those resources to buy fairly priced insurance is simply wasting money. Moreover, such an approach cannot provide anywhere near universal coverage. In the type of modeling described below, I find that even very generous subsidy policies cannot cover more than half of the uninsured on a voluntary basis. Indeed, some estimates suggest that subsidies focused solely on nongroup insurance could actually *raise* the number of uninsured through erosion of enrollment via employers that exceeds nongroup enrollment (Gruber 2006a).

---

3. Some of the attacks in the early 1990s on the Clinton plan were based on fears of restricted insurance choices.

Massachusetts: Synthesizing the Best of Both Ideas

The Commonwealth of Massachusetts is not typically regarded as a bastion of centrist thinking. While the state does have a strongly partisan Democratic legislature, at the time of reform in 2006, it had been led by Republican governors for fifteen years. Moreover, the particular Republican who was governor, Mitt Romney, laid out fundamental health care reform as one of the major goals for his administration. In addition, there was a very sophisticated and experienced advocacy community in Massachusetts that had been lobbying for universal coverage for years. This advocacy community was not ostracized but rather was well integrated and respected by the policymaking community.

Massachusetts also has three other advantages that made universal coverage more than just wishful thinking. First, the state has a relatively low uninsurance rate of about 11 percent of the nonelderly, compared to 18 percent nationally (Employee Benefit Research Institute 2007). This implies that fewer subsidies would be required to move to universal coverage. This lower insurance rate partly reflects the much higher rate of employer insurance offered in Massachusetts relative to the rest of the nation.

Second, there was a large federal transfer to the state at stake. As part of a section 1115 waiver to its Medicaid program that began in 1997, the state was receiving a large intergovernmental transfer from the federal government, which arose from matching funds for state transfers to safety net hospitals. In 2004–05 the Centers for Medicare and Medicaid Services (CMS) under the Bush administration was working to crack down on such intergovernmental transfers as a means of reducing federal spending. They also threatened to remove the Massachusetts intergovernmental transfer. In response the Romney administration suggested to the CMS that if the money continued to flow, it would be transitioned from payments to safety net providers toward subsidies to individuals to buy insurance. The CMS agreed to consider this alternative, imposing an early 2006 deadline on the state to present a plan to use the funds to increase insurance coverage or lose them altogether. This was a time bomb that had a substantial effect on state deliberations.

Finally, Massachusetts already had a ready-made funding source in place: the state uncompensated care pool. As part of an attempt at health care reform in the late 1980s, the state set up a mechanism through which hospitals were able to bill to the state the costs of treating low-income patients rather than absorbing those costs and passing them on to other payers. (Hospitals are forbidden from billing anyone who is pool eligible.) This pool had risen to more than $500 million by 2005. Since universal coverage would reduce the ranks of the uninsured, it would make a pool of this size unnecessary. Thus some of these funds could be rededicated to paying for a universal coverage system.

The Structure of Reform

The reform ultimately crafted and passed almost unanimously by the Massachusetts legislature has several key features.

PRIVATIZED PUBLIC INSURANCE FOR LOW-INCOME RESIDENTS. For adults whose income is less than three times the poverty line, a new program was established (Commonwealth Care Health Insurance Program, or "Commonwealth Care") that provides insurance coverage at subsidized rates. The legislation specifies that insurance must be free for adults who are below the poverty line, with minimal copayments of any type, and that it must be subsidized for adults with incomes between 100 and 300 percent of the poverty line, with copayments but no deductibles allowed. The exact subsidy levels and benefits were not prescribed other than by mandating that all insurance continue to include state-mandated benefits. Individuals were to choose from one of four Medicaid managed care organizations, the largest two of which were maintained by the large safety net hospitals.

NEW AND IMPROVED INSURANCE MARKET. There were also major changes to improve the insurance market. First, the nongroup and small group markets were merged to create one large market with guaranteed issue (that is, insurers must sell to all applicants) and community rating with a 2 to 1 age band (that is, insurers cannot differentiate prices across applicants by any factor other than age, and even then the ratio of prices for the oldest to youngest can only be 2 to 1). Second, the Connector was established as a clearinghouse for individuals to purchase private health insurance. The Connector has no monopoly power, and plans sold inside the Connector must be sold for the same price outside the Connector. It operates as somewhat of a market maker, however, specifying benefits packages that are likely to be emulated elsewhere. In a sense, the Connector operates as the anchor store in the mall, if the "mall" is the merged small group–nongroup market.

MANDATES. The law specified that all adults in the state must be covered by health insurance but only to the extent that such insurance was deemed "affordable" by the board of the Connector. Individuals who did not have coverage by December 31, 2007, would face the loss of their individual tax exemption (worth roughly $218), and those who did not have coverage in

2008 could be liable for a penalty of half of the premiums they would have paid if they had been insured. The law also mandated the charge of $295 per employee on all nonoffering employers with more than ten employees, and mandated that all employers with more than ten employees offer a section 125 account so that the employees could pay health insurance contributions with pretax dollars.

Within the context of this basic framework, the Connector board filled in a number of details around how the plan would work in Massachusetts, addressing questions such as, "What premiums should be charged for low-income residents in Commonwealth Care?" "What should define *minimum creditable coverage* for the purposes of qualifying for the insurance mandate?" "Is insurance affordable under the mandate? If not, who should be exempted from the mandate?"

To date, the reform in Massachusetts has been viewed as a success.[4] More than 300,000 of the state's 400,000 to 600,000 uninsured individuals were covered as of the end of 2007, despite the modest penalties in that year. The plans introduced through the Connector have been low priced, with options for young individuals at less than $150 a month and options for middle-aged persons at around $200 a month. Perhaps most important, all decisions have been made by consensus of the Connector board. This might be why advocacy groups of all stripes continue to be supportive of the evolving plan.

Taking Massachusetts National: The Details

A national version of the Massachusetts plan would follow this basic structure. At the same time, there are some limitations in the current structure (such as the restriction of subsidies to those below 300 percent of the poverty line) and some decisions made by the Connector board (such as the high rate of subsidization up to 300 percent of the poverty line) with which I disagree, and for which I make alternative proposals in this national plan.

Public Insurance

Public insurance entitlements would be frozen at their current level, which is typically around 200 percent of the poverty line for children in most states, and 100 percent of the poverty line for parents in many states. The federal government would continue to subsidize public expenditures by

---

4. Although, as one of the architects of the law and a member of the board overseeing its implementation, I am far from being an objective observer!

states through the Federal Medical Assistance Percentages or enhanced Federal Medical Assistance Percentages for those enrollees, with states paying the remainder.

Low-Income Pool

The remainder of low-income individuals in the United States who do not have access to employer-sponsored insurance (ESI) would be enrolled in new state-specific pools. Insurance companies would be eligible to offer insurance in these state-specific pools on a guaranteed issue basis. Within these pools, insurance prices would be completely community rated.

The benefits packages within the pools would vary based on income group. For the lowest-income individuals (those below the poverty line), coverage would be complete, with minimal cost sharing. As income increased, modest cost sharing would be introduced, reaching levels typical of the latest ESI offerings for the highest-income members of the pool (for example, a $20 copayment for physician visits or for prescriptions for generic drugs). There would be other cost controls in place, such as selective networks, to offset the more generous benefits provision for lower-income groups. In my modeling, I assume that the cost of insurance in this pool would equal the typical cost of insurance to large firms in each state, and that this would fall to 95 percent of that level for those between 100 and 200 percent of the poverty line, to 90 percent of that level for those between 200 and 300 percent, and to 85 percent of that level for those between 300 and 400 percent through cost sharing. In this way there is progressivity in both benefits design and in subsidies (detailed below, under " 'Universal Access' Plan"). There would also be redistribution across plans within this pool to offset cases with very high costs, with all insurers contributing to a fund going to offset part of the highest-cost patients. For example, insurers could pay an assessment as a share of premiums to finance a pool that can be tapped to help pay a share of the costs of any claim (or annual member costs) exceeding a given threshold.

Insurance would be subsidized in this pool by setting a limit as a share of income that individuals must pay for their insurance. These limits would be as follows:

—2 percent of income for those between 100 and 150 percent of the poverty line,

—4 percent of income for those between 150 and 200 percent of the poverty line,

—6 percent of income for those between 200 and 250 percent of the poverty line,

—8 percent of income for those between 250 and 300 percent of the poverty line,

—10 percent of income for those between 300 and 350 percent of the poverty line, and

—12 percent of income for those between 350 and 400 percent of the poverty line.

For comparison purposes, median income in the United States is between three and four times the poverty line, depending on family structure, so this schedule would subsidize insurance up to median income levels.

A problem with this approach is that low-income individuals who are charged high contributions for their ESI would have no way to afford them. This leads to serious equity concerns between those who do and those who do not have access to the subsidized pool. To address this, I propose to use the voucher approach that is part of the Massachusetts legislation (but which has not yet been implemented) and that is part of Governor Schwarzenegger's proposal in California. Under this approach, individuals who are offered ESI and who have incomes below 400 percent of the poverty line can come to the low-income pool but only if they bring with them their employer contribution toward health insurance to offset state costs. Employers are required to allow their employees to take their contributions with them.

Middle- and High-Income Pools

For many middle-income and all high-income families (above 400 percent of poverty), states would set up a new pooling mechanism, HealthMart, which would replace the existing nongroup insurance market. There would be a separate HealthMart in each state. HealthMart would be guaranteed issue, and there would be no health rating, although insurers could age rate on a basis of 3 to 1 (for example, the premiums for the oldest enrollees can be no more than three times the premiums for the youngest enrollees). Once again, any insurer participating in HealthMart would contribute toward a risk pool that offsets part of the costs of the highest-cost cases.

While HealthMart would replace the nongroup market, firms would also be allowed to buy into HealthMart, although if they did so, they could not offer their employees any non-HealthMart source of insurance (to avoid sending the worst risks to the HealthMart). For my microsimulation purposes, I do not model firms as leaving the existing group market to buy through HealthMart. By focusing just on nongroup purchasers, I will understate the reach of HealthMart, but it is difficult to project how attractive this option would be to employers.

HealthMart would offer three levels of benefits, and every participating insurer would have to offer all levels of benefits to avoid cream skimming. The highest level would be comparable to a low-copayment HMO today. The middle level would have an actuarial value of roughly 80 percent of that level, comparable to a typical plan newly offered by small firms in the United States. The bottom level would have an actuarial value of roughly 60 percent of that level. In Massachusetts, the minimum creditable coverage that forms this lower level features the following:

—a maximum deductible of $2,000 per individual or $4,000 per family,

—maximum out-of-pocket limits of $5,000 per individual or $10,000 per family,

—coverage of physician, hospital, mental health, and prescription drugs (but no coverage of dental or vision),

—at least three covered physician visits (at a copayment) before the deductible applies, and

—generic drugs covered with no deductible.

Critics have labeled such plans "underinsurance," but this is not consistent with available evidence. Health economics research has clearly shown that insurance can be more restrictive than the typical insurance package held today without having a negative impact on health. The famous RAND Health Insurance Experiment (Newhouse and the Insurance Experiment Group 1996), which I summarized in a report for the Kaiser Family Foundation (Gruber 2006b), showed clearly that for the average person, the copayments for medical care could rise significantly without health deteriorating. At the same time, there were some subgroups of ill patients for whom higher copayments did deter needed care—in particular, low-income ill patients. Exempting prevention and maintenance from the deductible in this way met the needs of this group, although ultimately a better solution would be to move toward treatment-specific copayments, along the lines suggested by Fendrick and others (2001).

While the plan above is not so different from plans offered by many insurers today, eventually an even better approach would be to move to the kind of income-related out-of-pocket limit advocated by Furman (2007).[5] This plan, in which individuals pay half their health care costs until they reach 7.5 percent of income, allows for strong income protection while making individuals price sensitive over a large range of their health spending.

5. See also Furman, chapter 7 in this volume.

Individual Mandate

Finally, all individuals in the United States would be required to purchase health insurance. This individual mandate would be enforced through the tax code. All individuals would be issued forms acknowledging their health insurance coverage; these forms could be attached to tax forms (as with W-2 forms). Any individual who does not have insurance would be assessed a fine equal to the cost of insurance for that individual. The monies collected from such fines would be a source of financing for the residual care pool.

A major issue with a mandate is affordability. As detailed in Gruber (2007), the share of income contributed by those who are below 400 percent of the poverty line under the schedule above is affordable for almost all individuals. For those above 400 percent of poverty line, the government would set an affordability limit of 15 percent of income. If the cost of the bottom-level plan exceeds this level for any individual or family, then the government would subsidize the difference to bring them to that level. These subsidies would be applied ex post through a tax rebate for individuals who have exceptionally high medical costs.

An important question for dynamic analysis of this type of proposal is how both the subsidy levels and the affordability limit evolve with the inevitable rapid rise in health care costs.

The Impacts: Microsimulation Results

To assess the impacts of a plan such as this, I turn to a microsimulation model that I have developed to model the effects of government intervention in insurance markets on insurance coverage and public sector costs. This model allows the user to input a set of policy parameters and to output the impact of that policy on public sector costs and the distribution of insurance coverage. This modeling approach is similar to that used by the Treasury Department, the CBO, and other government entities. It draws on the best evidence available in the health economics literature to model how individuals will respond to the changes in the insurance environment induced by changes in government policy. Gruber (2005) describes the model in detail.

It is important to highlight that the behavioral assumptions embedded in this model are based on the existing literature, which in turn derives estimates based on observed changes in prices and other insurance market characteristics. The plan I am modeling here is well beyond anything that has been implemented in U.S. insurance markets, so this is an out-of-sample prediction. While there is no strong basis for incorporating systematic changes in behavioral assumptions for this type of reform relative to past changes, the range of uncertainty around these behavioral assumptions is higher than for modeling more modest reforms.

Another issue that is not fully addressed here is the coverage of undocumented immigrants to the United States. For the purposes of this modeling, I assume that all individuals in the country will be able to access subsidies and will be subject to the mandate. To the extent that these assumptions are not true for undocumented immigrants, I am overstating the cost and reach of the proposal.

"Universal Access" Plan

I begin by analyzing a version of the plan that has subsidies and market reform but no individual mandate. It is important to highlight a key assumption of this model: that market reform can work effectively in the absence of a mandate. There is a significant concern that this will not be the case, as noted earlier. That is, if the government tries to impose the market reforms described above without a mandate, it will lead to rapidly rising prices and potentially even to a death spiral in insurance markets. I do not model this possibility, but there are real risks that it could arise.

The results of this analysis are presented in table 5-1. Panel 1 shows the distribution of insurance coverage, panel 2 shows federal government expenditures, and panel 3 shows the distribution of net (of tax changes) federal spending. Column 1 shows baseline values. All dollar figures are for year 2007 and are expressed in 2007 dollars.

This policy reduces the number of uninsured in the United States by 23 million. The increase in the pool, 53 million persons, minus the decrease in public insurance, 7 million persons, means that 46 million additional persons receive some federal subsidy. Comparing the 46 million persons receiving new subsidies to the 23 million–person reduction in the number of uninsured suggests that the rate at which this policy crowds out private purchase is roughly 50 percent. Note that this crowd-out represents net new federal spending, the large majority of which goes to help families who earn up to 200 percent of the poverty line pay for health insurance. Thus it may be considered a desirable feature by policymakers who care about more than achieving the maximum insured increase per new dollar spent.

This policy covers less than half of the total stock of uninsured, despite these generous subsidies and the comprehensive reform. This reflects the fact that many uninsured are not interested in obtaining coverage even at

Table 5-1. Alternative Approaches to Expand Insurance Coverage Results for the Nonelderly and Nondisabled

Units as indicated

Categories	(1) Baseline values[a]	(2) No mandate, no finance	(3) Mandate, no finance	(4) Mandate, remove exclusion	(5) Mandate, neutral financing[b]
Panel 1: Distribution of insurance coverage (millions of persons)					
Employer insured	160	144	153	136	136
Nongroup insured	11	4	5	4	4
Public	28	21	25	25	25
New pool	0	53	62	78	78
Uninsured	47	24	1	1	1
Panel 2: Federal government expenditures (billions of 2007 dollars)					
Public insurance (nonelderly/disabled)	58	43	50	50	50
Low-income subsidies	0	127	147	165	165
Income tax revenues on nonelderly	721	727	724	834	799
Payroll tax revenues on nonelderly	597	602	601	677	677
Net federal revenues	1,260	1,159	1,128	1,296	1,261
Change in net federal cost	. . .	101	131	−36	−1
Change in net state cost	. . .	−12	−7	−14	−14
Panel 3: Distribution of net federal spending (billions of 2007 dollars)					
Less than poverty line	. . .	50	63	63	63
One to two times poverty line	. . .	39	49	43	43
Two to three times poverty line	. . .	14	20	0	0
Three to four times poverty line	. . .	1	2	−28	0
Four to five times poverty line	. . .	−1	0	−28	−21
More than five times poverty line	. . .	−3	−2	−87	−87

Source: Author's calculations. For a complete description of the model, see Gruber (2005).

a. As of 2007.

b. Neutral financing via transitional tax credits for those with incomes between three and five times the poverty line. See text.

very high subsidy rates. Although this is clearly an out-of-sample prediction, this result is consistent with the large number of uninsured who are eligible for free public insurance but who do not enroll, as well as the large number of uninsured who are eligible for highly subsidized employer-provided insurance but who do not enroll. Universal access does not lead to anywhere near universal coverage.

At the same time, there is a large shift in where people get insurance. The number of individuals with ESI falls by 16 million under this scenario. Although this may seem like a large number, it is actually only 10 percent of the 160 million people who have ESI today. There is a much larger decline in the nongroup market, which shrinks by 7 million persons, or more than half. The new HealthMart pool increases by 53 million persons, which is more than both of these declines combined. The annual (fully phased-in) costs of this policy are presented in panel 2 of the table. The baseline costs, such as $58 billion in public insurance (federal Medicaid) expenditures, are low relative to numbers typically used, since my calculations focus only on the nonelderly and nondisabled. Similarly, the tax revenues apply only to the nonelderly.

This plan induces a modest reduction in traditional public insurance spending and a modest increase in income and payroll tax revenues. At the same time, there is a large new expenditure on the low-income subsidies to those in the pool (with a small share of those expenditures arising from the 15 percent cap on premiums for those above 400 percent of the poverty line). On net, the federal government spends $101 billion a year on this program. State governments save about $12 billion a year in lower public insurance expenditures and higher taxes.

The distributional implications of this policy are shown in panel 3. The policy is targeted, with virtually all of the benefits accruing to those below three times the poverty line. The benefits are negative at higher-income levels because lower levels of ESI imply higher wages and therefore higher tax payments.

"Universal Coverage" Plan

Column 3 shows the results for the same schedule of subsidies but includes the individual mandate, converting this plan from "universal access" to "universal coverage." This change has a number of noticeable effects on the results. First, the plan provides nearly universal coverage (once again, by assumption of a very effective mandate).[6] Second, there is much smaller erosion in ESI because the decline due to the availability of subsidies is off-set by increased enrollment among those eligible, previously uninsured, who are now mandated to get coverage. Similarly, there is a much smaller reduction in the number on public insurance. On net, 59 million persons receive new federal subsidies, compared with a 46 million–person reduction in the uninsured, for a crowd-out rate of only 28 percent.

The net federal cost of this plan is higher, at $131 billion. What is striking here, though, is that there is a 30 percent increase in cost for a more

---

6. I model the mandate by running the universal access version of the model, where individuals make voluntary choices, and then imposing that 95 percent of the remaining uninsured obtain coverage because they are mandated to do so.

than doubling of incremental insurance coverage. In part this reflects the fact that the newly insured through the mandate are somewhat healthier than those who signed up with the new subsidies without the mandate, but for the most part, this reflects that mandated individuals are largely unsubsidized. In this sense, the mandate forces most of those without insurance to pay for their coverage.

Financing the Plan: Removing the Tax Subsidy to ESI

A new $131 billion-a-year federal expenditure would place a strain on a federal budget that is already stretched thin to pay for other domestic and foreign initiatives. A natural source of financing for this initiative is available, however: the tax subsidy to ESI. While wages received are taxed, employer expenditures on health insurance received are not. Thus individuals receive a large tax break by not being taxed on a particular form of their compensation.

This large subsidy to ESI is regressive since it is worth the most to the higher-income individuals with the highest tax rates (and since higher-income individuals are more likely to be insured and to have insurance that is more expensive). In addition, this subsidy to ESI induces inefficient insurance purchase since individuals can buy excessively generous insurance with pretax dollars. Of course, in the absence of any other pooling mechanism for workers, the ESI tax subsidy may be a necessary price to pay to keep the ESI market intact. With a new pooling mechanism, however, reductions in ESI are not problematic. It does not matter whether or not individuals obtain insurance through employers as long as they have access to some group insurance mechanism.

In addition, the tax subsidy to ESI has a major advantage over other sources of financing, in that it ensures that the health plan will continue to be paid for, into the future. Since the savings from repealing the tax exclusion rise at the same rate as health care costs, a health plan funded through this mechanism would be covered in each year of its operation. Any other source of financing, such as taxes on high-income earners, would only rise at the rate of the economy. With health care costs rising more quickly than the economy, these alternative sources of financing would eventually fall short of the revenue needed to finance the plan into the future.

I therefore consider the impact of funding the national Massachusetts plan by removing this tax subsidy. More specifically, employer expenditures on health insurance would be included in taxable wages for individuals. An important issue to resolve with such a policy is whether ESI expenditures would be included for both income and payroll tax purposes and, if included for both, whether the resulting revenues would be dedicated to the social insurance programs financed by these payroll taxes or recaptured for use in funding the universal coverage plan.

The results of incorporating this financing are presented in column 4 of table 5-1. There is now a substantial disruption to employer-provided insurance, with coverage in this market falling by about 15 percent. This represents roughly 32 million persons who either lose ESI due to firms no longer offering coverage or switch from ESI to the subsidized low-income pool, and about 8 million persons who move onto ESI due to the mandate. In these cases wages rise by an amount equal to the reduction in health insurance outlays, and affected individuals use those extra wages to pay for health insurance through the new pool. The changes in public and non-group insurance are similar to column 2, while the new pool has grown to 78 million persons. Once again it is important to highlight that this is an attempt to use a model based on historical experience to predict a major new policy change, so there is considerable uncertainty around these estimates. In particular, if removing the ESI exclusion changes the entire equilibrium in the insurance market, there could be a race to the bottom: firms might stop providing insurance more broadly.

The impact on government expenditures and tax revenues is shown in panel 2 of column 4. The costs of the low-income subsidies have risen from $147 billion in the case of no financing to $165 billion a year with financing, since the size of the low-income pool expands. At the same time, there is a $110 billion rise in income tax revenues and a $76 billion increase in payroll tax revenues. Therefore, if all of these tax revenue increases were dedicated to financing the plan, there would be a net federal surplus of $36 billion (even ignoring the $14 billion net gain to the states).

Of course, such a policy would have large distributional consequences. The spending would be targeted to the lower parts of the income distribution while the higher taxes would be borne by higher-income groups. In fact, while there would be substantial gains for those below two times the federal poverty line, there would be losses at three or more times the federal poverty line. (Median income in the United States is between three to four times the poverty line, depending on family structure.) Thus such a policy would be a net loser for more than half the families in the United States.

In principle, however, the extra tax revenues raised by this policy could be used to help cover the losses to those with income below five times the poverty line. Most directly (if not politically realistically), we could introduce a transitional tax credit to assist those who are at between three and five times the poverty line who would be disadvantaged by this change. This credit would be equal to $380 per individual and $950 per family for those between 300 and 400 percent of the poverty line, and would fall to $120 per individual and $300 per family for those between 400 and 500 percent of the poverty line. Column 5 shows that adding such a credit ("neutral financing") would lead to no net losses for those with incomes between three and four times the poverty line, and compared to the policy without the tax credit, would reduce by 25 percent the losses to those with incomes between four and five times the poverty line. Thus, by recycling revenues, the United States could finance universal coverage in a way where there are net gains to all income classes below the median.

Conclusion

The political and economic environment in the United States is more favorable for universal health insurance coverage now than it has been for several decades. States are moving aggressively toward universal coverage, and many are advocating that the federal government follow suit. In this chapter, I have laid out one approach to universal coverage that both guarantees affordable coverage for all Americans and is consistent with market principles by relying on private insurance markets. Such a plan is working in Massachusetts and can work for the nation as a whole.

It is important to note that there are principally two problems with the health care system in America: a lack of coverage and poor cost-effectiveness. The health industry knows how to solve the first problem but not how to solve the second. There is important ongoing research about cost-effectiveness, which is measured as quality of care relative to cost of care, including geographic variation in health care spending and the cost-saving potential of electronic medical records. This type of research should continue, but we should not hold uninsurance—a problem that we know how to solve—hostage to a problem that we do not know how to solve.

References

Congressional Budget Office (CBO). 2003. "How Many People Lack Health Insurance and for How Long?" CBO paper (May).

Currie, Janet, and Jonathan Gruber. 1996a. "Health Insurance Eligibility, Utilization of Medical Care, and Child Health." *Quarterly Journal of Economics* 111, no. 2: 431–66.

————. 1996b. "Saving Babies: The Efficacy and Cost of Recent Expansions of Medicaid Eligibility for Pregnant Women." *Journal of Political Economy* 104, no. 6: 1263–96.

Employee Benefit Research Institute. 2007. "Sources of Health Insurance and Characteristics of the Uninsured: Analysis of the March 2007 Current Population Survey." Issue Brief 310. Washington (October).

Fendrick, A. Mark, and others. 2001. "A Benefit-Based Copay for Prescription Drugs: Patient Contribution Based on Total Benefits, Not Drug Acquisition Costs." *American Journal of Managed Care* 7, no. 9: 861–67.

Furman, Jason. 2007. "The Promise of Progressive Cost Consciousness in Health Care Reform." Discussion Paper 2007-05. Brookings, Hamilton Project (April).

Gruber, Jonathan. 2001. "Health Insurance and the Labor Market." In *The Handbook of Health Economics*, edited by Joseph Newhouse and Anthony Culyer, pp. 645–706. Amsterdam: North Holland.

————. 2005. "Tax Policy for Health Insurance." In *Tax Policy and the Economy 19*, edited by James Poterba, pp. 39–63. MIT Press.

————. 2006a. "The Cost and Coverage Impact of the President's Health Insurance Budget Proposals." Report. Washington: Center on Budget and Policy Priorities (February).

————. 2006b. "The Role of Consumer Copayments for Health Care: Lessons from the RAND Health Insurance Experiment and Beyond." Report. Menlo Park, Calif.: Kaiser Family Foundation (October).

————. 2007. "Evidence on Affordability from Consumer Expenditures and Employee Enrollment in Employer-Sponsored Health Insurance." MIT.

Gruber, Jonathan, and Brigitte C. Madrian. 2004. "Health Insurance, Labor Supply, and Job Mobility: A Critical Review of the Literature." In *Health Policy and the Uninsured*, edited by Catherine McLaughlin, pp. 97–178. Washington: Urban Institute Press.

Hanratty, Maria. 1996. "Canadian National Health Insurance and Infant Health." *American Economic Review* 86, no. 1: 276–84.

Institute of Medicine (IOM). 2001. *Coverage Matters: Insurance and Health Care.* Washington.

Lurie, Nicole, and others. 1984. "Termination from Medi-Cal: Does It Affect Health?" *New England Journal of Medicine* 311, no. 7: 480–84.

Madrian, Brigitte C. 1994. "Employment-Based Health Insurance and Job Mobility: Is There Evidence of Job Lock?" *Quarterly Journal of Economics* 109, no. 1: 27–54.

Newhouse, Joseph P., and the Insurance Experiment Group. 1996. *Free For All? Lessons from the RAND Health Insurance Experiment.* Harvard University Press.

Nichols, Len, Jonathan Gruber, and Mark V. Pauly. 2007. "Health Debate Reality Check: The Role of Individual Requirements." Policy brief. Washington: New America Foundation (December).

Woolhandler, Steffie, Terry Campbell, and David U. Himmelstein. 2003. "Costs of Health Care Administration in the United States and Canada." *New England Journal of Medicine* 349, no. 8: 768–75.

Mending the Medicare Prescription Drug Benefit

Improving Consumer Choices and Restructuring Purchasing

6

RICHARD G. FRANK AND JOSEPH P. NEWHOUSE

Prescription drugs play an increasingly central role in health care delivery, accounting for about 12 percent of personal health care spending in 2006.[1] They are critical in managing many chronic diseases and meeting other health needs of the elderly. Yet the original Medicare program, the main federal health care program for the elderly, did not cover most outpatient prescription drugs. In making this choice, Medicare simply followed the lead of the private health insurance plans that existed at its creation in the 1960s, when the clinical importance of drugs was much smaller than it is today.

As a result, at the turn of the twenty-first century, Medicare recipients either paid for most drugs themselves or relied on a patchwork of financing arrangements. Twenty-five percent of them had no drug coverage during the entire year, and as many as 40 percent had no coverage for some part

We are grateful to Ernst Berndt, Jason Bordoff, Arnold Epstein, Leif Haase, Judith Lave, Tom McGuire, Dan Mendelson, Tricia Neuman, Robert Reischauer, Judy Wagner, and Gail Wilensky for helpful comments, although, of course, they do not necessarily agree with our conclusions and are not responsible for any errors. Sam Kina provided expert research assistance.
1. Centers for Medicare and Medicaid Services, "National Health Expenditure Accounts, 2006," table 2 (www.cms.hhs.gov/NationalHealthExpendData/downloads/tables.pdf).

of the year (Holtz-Eakin 2003; Congressional Budget Office [CBO] 2002).[2] About 11 percent relied on an individually purchased private plan to pay for drugs, and the remainder relied on either Medicaid (16 percent), health maintenance organizations (14 percent), employer-provided retiree coverage (30 percent), or other publicly financed programs (4 percent) (CBO 2002).

In 1999 the average Medicare beneficiary used $1,250 worth of prescription drugs, paying for 38 percent of that amount out of pocket (CBO 2002). Some spent much more: the CBO estimated that in 2005 about 17 percent of Medicare recipients spent $5,000 or more on such drugs. Meanwhile many of the less affluent elderly bore a particularly heavy burden: the 48 percent of Medicare beneficiaries with incomes between 100 and 300 percent of the federal poverty line were less likely to have any prescription drug coverage than those with higher incomes. (Most of the elderly below the poverty line were covered by Medicaid.) On average this lower-income group paid 43 percent of their drug costs out of pocket (Holtz-Eakin 2003).

Besides putting many elderly Americans at serious financial risk, the absence of insurance coverage for prescription drugs resulted in many elderly persons failing to get appropriate treatment for major chronic illnesses such as congestive heart failure and diabetes.[3] This may well have added more to Medicare spending for hospital and physician services than the drugs themselves would have cost. For all these reasons, in the early years of the new century, Congress faced mounting pressure to add a prescription drug benefit to the Medicare program.

In 2003, after a long and contentious debate, Congress passed and President George W. Bush signed the Medicare Modernization Act (MMA), which provided prescription drug coverage under a new Part D of Medicare. The new program embodied several important policy features, some of them controversial. Congress decided to give beneficiaries in traditional Medicare a choice among stand-alone competing prescription drug plans (PDPs) rather than the single, government-administered program, or traditional Medicare, that most beneficiaries use for hospital and physician services. Beneficiaries enrolled in Medicare Advantage, however, would receive their new drug benefit through their Advantage plan. Congress also

---

2. The 40 percent estimate is based on CBO's analysis of the Medicare Current Beneficiary Survey 1999.

3. Dana G. Safran and others, "Prescription Drug Coverage and Seniors: Findings from a 2003 National Survey," *Health Affairs*, web exclusive, April 19, 2005 (content. healthaffairs.org/cgi/content/abstract/hlthaff.w5.152v1).

Box 6-1. Medicare, Part D, and the Federal Budget

In 2006 Medicare and Medicaid together accounted for 21 percent of federal outlays (net of receipts for Medicare) and 4.1 percent of GDP (according to the CBO March 2008 baseline).[1] If historical growth rates of spending persist in both health care and the federal budget, by 2016 these programs will account for 32 percent of the federal budget and 6.8 percent of GDP. Under the more optimistic assumption that health care will grow at a rate only 1 percentage point above growth in GDP, by 2016 Medicare and Medicaid would still account for about 30 percent of the federal budget and 6.5 percent of GDP (calculations based on CBO 2006b and 2007). Thus the growth of Medicare and Medicaid will continue to place enormous strains on the budget.

The Part D benefit added claims of $49 billion to Medicare outlays in 2007, equivalent to 11 percent of total (gross) outlays for that year. By 2018 Part D is projected to account for 15 percent of outlays. Thus cost-effective purchasing is important to the financial health of the program, and it is critical to consider the balance of where the burden of paying for drugs rests.

1. For federal outlays and GDP, see Congressional Budget Office, "Summary Table 1: CBO's Baseline Budget Outlook" (www.cbo.gov/ftpdocs/89xx/doc8917/Summary.4.1.shtml#1070888); for Medicare, see "CBO's March 2008 Baseline: Medicare" (www.cbo.gov/budget/factsheets/2008b/medicare.pdf); and for Medicaid, see "Fact Sheet for CBO's March 2008 Baseline: Medicaid" (www.cbo.gov/budget/factsheets/2008b/medicaidBaseline.pdf).

---

decided against using administered prices such as traditional Medicare applies to almost all other services. In fact, the MMA prohibits government from being directly involved in price negotiations for prescription drugs purchased under Part D. Instead prices are set in negotiations between PDPs, which are mostly owned by pharmacy benefit management companies [PBMs] or health insurance companies, and drug manufacturers.

These policy choices, along with the chosen design for cost sharing between beneficiaries and plans (described below), were made against the background of a federal budget projected to run substantial deficits far into the future, and a Medicare program forecast to grow from 2.5 percent of GDP in 2003 to 4.4 percent in 2016 under current law (CBO 2006b; see also box 6-1). Congress also set an explicit limit of $400 billion for the forecast ten-year federal cost (2004–13) of Part D. Figure 6-1 shows spending projections for Medicare with and without Part D, based on the March 2006 CBO forecasts. Cumulative spending projections now total $846 billion for 2008–17, in part because the budget window has shifted forward: the years 2004 and 2005, when the program was not in effect, have been replaced by 2014 and 2015, when it is, and inflation tends to increase nominal costs as one moves further out in time.[4]

---

4. CBO, "CBO's March 2008 Baseline: Medicare" (www.cbo.gov/budget/factsheets/2008b/medicare.pdf).

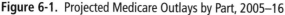

Figure 6-1. Projected Medicare Outlays by Part, 2005–16

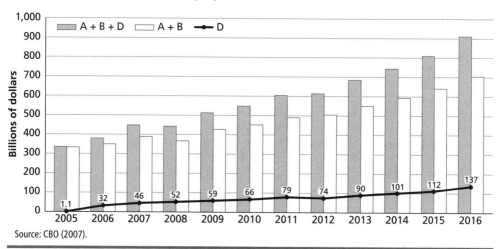

Source: CBO (2007).

In its brief existence to date, Part D has succeeded in providing afford-able prescription drug coverage to millions of elderly Medicare recipients for the first time. Approximately 2.7 million low-income Medicare bene-ficiaries have obtained comprehensive coverage for prescription drugs where previously they had none.[5] These are very important benefits. Pub-lic opinion about the program overall has been quite positive, but it also points to areas where improvements may be warranted. A Kaiser Family Foundation–Harvard School of Public Health poll (Kaiser Family Foun-dation 2006b) reports that 76 percent of respondents enrolled in a Part D plan had either very positive or somewhat positive views of their plan, and 72 percent said that Part D overall was helpful or very helpful to them. At the same time, however, 75 percent reported that the program was "too complicated," and 60 percent favored reducing the number of plan choices offered.

Although the program's cost for the next ten years (2008–17) is now more than double the cost expected for the first ten years (2004–13), the premiums offered by PDPs to Part D recipients have been on average lower than the CBO and others had initially projected (CBO 2004). The reasons

5. Juliette Cubanski and Patricia Neuman, "Status Report on Medicare Part D Enroll-ment in 2006: Analysis of Plan-Specific Market Share and Coverage," *Health Affairs*, web exclusive, November 21, 2006 (content.healthaffairs.org/webexclusives/index.dtl?year= 2006).

are somewhat speculative but may relate to the lack of any previous experience with a prescription drug benefit designed like Part D. Also, the number of plans participating in Part D far exceeded projections, generating more price competition than expected, and Part D in practice relied far less on specially constituted "fallback" plans than had been forecast—in fact, fallback plans were not resorted to at all. Moreover, the cost projections were based on the 1999–2000 Medicare Current Beneficiary Survey and Centers for Medicare and Medicaid Services (CMS) projections of prescription drug spending; these projections were made during a time of very rapid spending increases, after which spending rises unexpectedly moderated. Finally, premiums may also have been lower than expected because the flow of unique drugs (those for which no therapeutic substitute exists) has dropped dramatically in the last few years, allowing for more competition among drugs.

The program's success in bringing prescription drug coverage to millions, at lower-than-expected costs to the participants, is most welcome. Yet the desire to design a program that would accomplish several important objectives at once—comprehensive coverage, reliance on private PDPs modeled on commercial PBMs, a wide choice of plans, and the use of market forces to establish prices, all within a $400 billion ten-year budget— led to some unfortunate policy choices. In what follows, we first briefly describe some of the problems that Part D has encountered and then offer some proposals to mend the program's flaws while preserving its achievements. The changes we propose apply only to the 80 percent of Medicare beneficiaries enrolled in traditional Medicare; we believe that those enrolled in Medicare Advantage who receive drug coverage through their plans, should they elect it, should continue in those arrangements. In that arrangement, plans have an incentive to structure the drug benefit, both formularies and cost sharing, to minimize all Medicare costs (that is, including Parts A and B), whereas PDPs have an incentive to minimize drug costs. These two different sets of incentives will generally not be similar.

Some Problematic Design Choices

A serious problem with Part D, as the respondents to the Kaiser Family Foundation–Harvard survey observed, is its complexity. Consider the array of plans now being offered under Part D to the elderly and disabled, many of whom have trouble negotiating complex choices. Although the MMA requires that each plan meet certain minimum standards (see below), each has considerable leeway in designing its formulary (the list of specific drugs covered). Each plan also has discretion in the terms of coverage it offers, such as copayments, prior authorization requirements, quantity limits, and requirements to try a lower-priced drug that is therapeutically similar before resorting to a more expensive one (sometimes referred to as step therapy or "fail first" requirements). Over thirty-six combinations of the program's key provisions alone are possible.

The result is that a large number of private PDPs that differ in important but often subtle ways are being offered to recipients of traditional Medicare across the nation. The actual number of plans differs from state to state and in 2007 ranged from forty-five in Alaska to sixty-six in Pennsylvania and West Virginia (Kaiser Family Foundation 2007). For an individual beneficiary, the dimension of the choice problem depends on the number and type of drugs he or she uses (the average Medicare beneficiary uses five different drugs). This complexity has potentially discouraged some enrollment, created confusion, and likely led to choices of coverage that are not cost effective (U.S. Government Accountability Office 2006; Medicare Payment Advisory Commission [MedPAC] 2006, McFadden 2006).

A second problem is that of adverse selection. The reliance on competition among PDPs creates strong incentives for PDPs to seek out those enrollees they believe they can serve at lowest cost while encouraging them to exclude others (Pauly and Zeng 2004). These incentives may lead PDPs to choose benefit structures, formulary designs, and drug utilization review processes so as to discourage enrollment by expected high-cost individuals. Both the MMA and the CMS, which administers the program, recognize this issue, and the law attempts to counter these incentives by providing for some adjustment in payments to plans for their varying mixes of risks. But existing risk adjustment technology can account for only a portion of the predictable differences in expected spending across plans. Wrobel and others (2003) show that the risk adjusters used by the CMS account for about 23 percent of the variance in drug spending per year among the elderly, or less than half of the total explainable variation of at least 55 percent. (Some variation, of course, is unexplainable.) Thus, even though PDPs are paid more for enrolling people with higher drug needs, strong incentives remain for them to enroll low-utilizing recipients, and the information needed to predict who will be a low-utilizing recipient is readily available.

Four more problems arise from other provisions of the law. First, competition keeps prices down only when there are competitors. Manufacturers of unique drugs face little or no competition, and makers of such drugs that are heavily used by the elderly can essentially name their price. We present below some evidence on how common this may be.

A second problem arises because some persons are eligible for both Medicare and Medicaid. Before Part D was enacted, Medicaid was already buying prescription drugs for its low-income participants under a "best price" rule: the price at which manufacturers must sell is the lower of the best private price or 15.1 percent below the average manufacturer price, the price at which manufacturers sell to wholesalers net of prompt-pay discounts (Scott-Morton 1997). The MMA shifted the responsibility for paying for prescription drugs for some 6.6 million dually eligible beneficiaries from Medicaid to Medicare. This appears to have resulted in significant price increases for drugs used by these beneficiaries, giving some drug manufacturers a windfall. AstraZeneca, Eli Lilly, Bristol-Myers Squibb, and Pfizer have acknowledged, in filings with the Securities and Exchange Commission, reductions in the size of rebates they have granted to Medicaid, implying that the prices they receive have increased.[6]

Third, in order to meet the ten-year budget target, Part D could not afford full coverage. Instead Congress created the notorious "doughnut hole," which leaves a coverage gap for each participant's total annual drug spending between $2,400 and $5,451 (in 2007). Part D "basic" plans are actually prohibited from increasing deductibles and reducing the size of the doughnut hole, even if doing so keeps the premium constant. The result is that the expected 25 percent of Part D enrollees who will incur at least $2,400 in drug costs in a given year will have to pay 100 percent of their next $3,051 of spending on drugs—this after having already absorbed substantial out-of-pocket spending on premiums, deductibles, and copayments for the first $2,400.[7] Although this design offers catastrophic coverage, in that most spending beyond the doughnut hole is covered, it runs counter to the fundamental insurance principle that emphasizes protection against

6. Neither the population covered nor cost sharing changed materially for the dually eligible, and therefore these factors cannot explain the rise in drug company revenue. See the 2006 Forms 6-K and 10-Q for AstraZeneca, Bristol-Myers Squibb, Eli Lilly, Glaxo-SmithKline, Merck, Novartis, Pfizer, and Wyeth, available at U.S. Securities and Exchange Commission, "SEC Filings and Forms (EDGAR)" (www.sec.gov/edgar.shtml).

7. See Juliette Cubanski and Patricia Neuman, "Status Report on Medicare Part D Enrollment in 2006: Analysis of Plan-Specific Market Share and Coverage," *Health Affairs*, web exclusive, November 21, 2006 (content.healthaffairs.org/webexclusives/index.dtl?year=2006).

Under the standardized benefit, cost sharing for those who spend enough to just reach the doughnut hole amounts to almost $800. This, of course, is in addition to cost sharing for physician visits, hospital stays, and other services.

larger risks (in this case, that of incurring drug expenses between $2,400 and $5,451) over smaller ones (that of incurring less than $2,400).

The doughnut hole feature of the Part D benefit design affects behavior in both desirable and less salutary ways. One recent analysis of enrollees in a large regional PDP found that people entering the doughnut hole increased their use of generic medications but some discontinued those medications used to treat chronic conditions (Borschow 2007). Thus the design encouraged economizing behavior via generic substitution but also led to medication discontinuities that may result in adverse health outcomes and higher spending for hospital and physician services.

Finally, before Part D's enactment, Medicare Part B already covered certain drugs, and Congress chose to leave these drugs under Part B rather than consolidate all coverage under the new Part D. The principal criterion for determining whether a drug is covered under Part B or Part D is how it is administered (broadly speaking, whether usually administered by a health professional or self-administered, respectively). As a result, manufacturers have an incentive to game the system, formulating the delivery mechanisms for new drugs so as to generate the greatest reimbursement.

Steps toward Mending the Drug Benefit

The enactment of a Medicare drug benefit was a major political accomplishment. But as we have just documented, the policy that was politically acceptable has numerous undesirable properties (see also Huskamp and others 2000). It is tempting to propose starting over, and many ideas have been offered for how to do that. But a radical change in the program's architecture at this point would require refashioning a delicate political compromise, which could endanger the gains that have been made. Starting over would also add to the confusion and frustration of the beneficiary population. Fortunately, important steps can be taken within the existing architecture of Part D to mend the program and improve its impact. We focus on four such steps: simplifying beneficiary choices, improving the benefit design and filling the doughnut hole, enhancing the purchasing power of PDPs and reducing costs to the government, and ending the confusing distinction between Part B and Part D drugs.

Better Informing Consumers and Simplifying Choices

Although many Americans under sixty-five have a choice of health plan, virtually none has an independent choice of a drug plan. For most people under sixty-five, drug coverage comes packaged with their employer-provided health insurance plan. (Indeed, even where a choice of health plan is offered, the employer may have carved out the drug benefit and given all the business to one PBM, in which case employees do not even have an indirect choice of drug plan.) The same used to be true for Medicare: before Part D, except for the small minority who purchased individual Medigap plans, Medicare beneficiaries with supplemental coverage for drugs through a prior employer had no choice of drug plan. Thus Part D presents Medicare beneficiaries with a very different setting for purchasing insurance against drug spending than had previously existed in the marketplace. (Most beneficiaries who have employer-provided retiree health insurance have continued with that coverage and thus do not face the situation we are about to describe.)

HOW PDP CHOICE WORKS. Under Part D the nation is divided into thirty-four geographic regions that define PDP markets. Within these markets PDPs may offer Medicare beneficiaries electing to participate in Part D a choice of three types of plans: a standardized benefit plan, a plan that is actuarially equivalent to the standardized benefit plan, or a plan that offers enhanced benefits.[8] In 2007 the standardized benefit plan consisted of a $265 deductible, 75 percent coverage (25 percent coinsurance) up to $2,400 in total spending, zero benefits between $2,400 and $5,451, and "catastrophic" coverage above $5,451. In the catastrophic range, which comes into effect after a total of $3,850 in out-of-pocket spending, beneficiaries with incomes over 150 percent of the poverty line pay either a 5 percent coinsurance or $2 per generic prescription ($5 per branded prescription), whichever is greater. (Cost sharing for those with incomes under 135 percent of the poverty line is nominal, and a sliding scale applies between 135 and 150 percent of the poverty level.) The dollar values for the deductible, coverage thresholds, and copayment obligations increase annually with growth in total Part D spending.

Each PDP may offer one actuarially equivalent plan design where deductibles, copayment and coinsurance arrangements, and the availability of mail order services vary. PDPs have considerable discretion in designing such benefits. For example, copayment arrangements frequently involve tiering, which means that the copayment varies according to the formulary status of the drug. Generics carry the lowest copayments, followed by preferred branded drugs, with nonpreferred branded drugs and so-called

---

8. Regulations limit the ways in which actuarial equivalence can be realized. Most significantly, plans that do not offer enhanced benefits cannot increase the deductible above that in the standardized plan.

Table 6-1. Distribution of Key Plan Features across Medicare Part D Plan Types, 2006 and 2007[a]

Feature	All plans	Percent of all plans with indicated feature		
		Standardized plans	Actuarially equivalent plans	Enhanced plans
Deductible				
Zero	60 (58)	. . .	(18)	(40)
Reduced	8	. . .	(5)	(3)
$250	32 (34)	9	(25)	(0)
Cost sharing				
25 percent copay	10 (9)	(9)	(0)	(0)
Tiered	90 (91)	. . .	(48)	(43)
Coverage in doughnut hole				
Generics only	27	. . .	(0)	(0)
Generics and branded	1	. . .	(0)	(2)
None	71	(9)	(48)	(27)
Memorandum: share of all plans	100	12 (9)	41 (48)	47 (43)

Source: Hoadley and others (2006).

a. 2006 values are shown in parentheses.

specialty tier drugs carrying the highest copayments. The definition of preferred branded drugs can differ substantially across plans. Each PDP may also offer one plan with enhanced benefits (such as coverage in the doughnut hole), but the premium for that plan must then reflect its full additional cost—Medicare will not subsidize coverage that is above the actuarial value of the basic benefit. Table 6-1 presents a distribution of plans by major benefit design features, illustrating the variety of choices available.

Across the thirty-four regions, a total of 1,875 drug plans were offered in 2007. Of these, 228 offered the standardized benefit, 760 offered benefits that were actuarially equivalent to the standardized benefit, and 887 plans offered enhanced benefits (Hoadley and others 2006). The bulk of beneficiaries are enrolled in plans offered by sixteen large PBMs or health insurance companies (MedPAC 2006). In each region, plans with sufficiently low premiums can qualify to receive low-income subsidies and accept people who are automatically enrolled because they are dually eligible for Medicare and Medicaid (see below). The number of such plans in each region currently ranges from five to twenty (Hoadley and others 2006).

As described above, PDPs also have some discretion over the formulary designs they offer. Before Part D went into effect, all PDPs were required to submit their proposed formulary design to the CMS for approval. This requirement was put in place to limit the ability of PDPs to use formulary design to compete for good risks and thereby discourage enrollment by Medicare beneficiaries with high expected levels of prescription drug spending. Administering this condition forced the CMS to determine whether a given plan's proposed breadth of coverage within particular therapeutic classes was adequate. This was a scientifically and economically complicated and difficult task. Because formularies involve choices among 1,000 or more major drugs, the potential number of acceptable formularies is quite large. In addition, PDPs can use a variety of management techniques that assist efficient prescribing but may also make their plans more or less attractive to certain beneficiaries. These techniques include prior authorization requirements, stepped care protocols, and fail-first policies, among others. These dimensions create numerous other permutations in the number and types of drugs that can be used to treat specific conditions, especially for people with multiple conditions.[9]

In short, Medicare beneficiaries in a typical region face a choice of roughly fifty different drug plans, including standardized benefit plans, actuarially equivalent plans, and enhanced plans. In choosing a plan, beneficiaries must make comparisons across the numerous features that distinguish one plan from another and must understand which features are most important to the management of their own drug needs. An important body of research documents that the typical consumer can become overwhelmed by such a large number of complicated choices (Camerer 2000; McFadden 2006; Thaler 1999). Although the CMS and other agencies have assisted beneficiaries in choosing plans, such complexity makes it likely that consumers will make important errors in choosing a PDP.

McFadden (2006) reports on a survey of older Americans undertaken in November 2005, just before the launch of the Part D benefit. Respondents were given a hypothetical choice among no drug coverage, the standardized plan, and three actuarially equivalent alternatives. Only about 36 percent of respondents chose a plan that offered them the best financial protection (that is, the lowest expected out-of-pocket costs). In fact, only 26 percent preferred the plan with the best catastrophic protection, even though it was the plan with the lowest out-of-pocket costs for 51 percent of respondents. These results are troubling because the

---

9. Formulary design and the use of other utilization management techniques are not part of the assessment of actuarial equivalence in benefit design.

choices studied by McFadden are far simpler than those actually faced by Medicare beneficiaries.[10]

Initial CMS data on Part D enrollment show that nearly 25 percent of Medicare recipients who were estimated to qualify for a low-income subsidy for drug coverage did not enroll in any Part D plan (Kaiser Family Foundation 2006a). This is a surprising result, given that coverage was essentially free to this population. The complexity of the decision may have discouraged enrollment among this group of Medicare recipients, who typically have less education than others and frequently live alone.

A survey conducted for MedPAC in February 2006 asked Medicare beneficiaries about their decisions to join a Part D plan. Most beneficiaries were aware of the benefit but expressed difficulty in understanding how it worked. They frequently relied on family members for help in choosing, but the family members, too, were generally poorly informed about the Part D benefit. The survey reported that 41 percent of those who signed up, 65 percent of those who considered signing up, and 28 percent of those who did not consider signing up found it either difficult or very difficult to understand the choices. The survey also asked those who did not enroll what their primary reason was for that decision. Among those without some other form of coverage, 36 percent said they did not fill many prescriptions, 9 percent said they were too confused, 7 percent did not know enough to join, and 24 percent thought the program would not save them much money (MedPAC 2006). It is not clear whether this pattern of responses is what would be observed with the introduction of any new product, or whether it reflects the complex structure of choices within Part D specifically. The additional enrollment experience gained during 2007 will allow further understanding of this issue.

A recent study of PDP premiums shows that, holding benefit design and formulary structure constant, premiums were not lower in markets with more plan offerings (Simon and Lucarelli 2006). The study also finds only a weak relationship between expected out-of-pocket costs (a measure of plan generosity) and the premium charged. A possible explanation of the latter finding is that expected out-of-pocket costs may vary considerably depending on how the beneficiary's drugs are classified on the plan's formulary. But one plausible interpretation consistent with both findings is that the choice environment is so complex that consumers cannot effec-

---

10. Ironically, however, the weaker the ability of consumers to make effective choices between plans, the less of a problem adverse selection poses.

tively respond to market signals, and thus the expected relationships among prices, choice, and product characteristics either do not hold or hold only weakly.

There is as yet no direct evidence on PDP responses to selection incentives. The June 2006 MedPAC report suggests that it may be too early to tell how benefit structure, utilization management, and formulary design tools will be used and what their ultimate impact on enrollment patterns will be.

IMPROVING THE PLAN CHOICE PROCESS. Clearly, Part D benefits confront participants with a far more complex set of options than people face in most employment-based health insurance programs. We believe that their choices could be reduced and simplified without harming price competition among PDPs.[11] Indeed, simplification of choice would most likely result in more effective consumer choice and enhanced competition.

Choices can be made simpler and clearer by developing a set of standardized benefit packages within the groups of actuarially equivalent and enhanced PDPs and reducing the number of choices within each grouping, including the existing standardized plan. During 2006 the CMS floated the notion of reducing the number of plans being offered under Part D, because of concerns about confusion. But in fact the number of PDPs offered increased by 31 percent in 2007 (Hoadley and others 2006).

Benefit standardization has already proved effective in health insurance for the elderly, in the so-called Medigap market where Medicare recipients can purchase supplemental insurance. The aims of standardization for Part D parallel those originally pursued in regulating the Medigap market (Rice and Thomas 1992). The Baucus amendments to the Omnibus Budget Reconciliation Act of 1990 stated that Medigap plans must "provide benefits that offer consumers the ability to purchase the benefits that are [currently] available in the market [and] balance the objectives of (i) simplifying the market to facilitate comparisons among policies, (ii) avoiding adverse selection, (iii) providing consumer choice, (iv) providing market stability, and promoting competition" (P.L. 96-265, sec. 507).

The 1990 legislation required that Medigap plans conform to one of ten standardized plans. The National Association of Insurance Commissioners (NAIC) was assigned the task of developing the standardized plans (Fox,

---

11. Research on the impact on price competition as choices increase shows that, after four or five competitors are present, additional entry offers little in the way of additional price reductions (Bresnahan and Reiss 1991). Reiffen and Ward (2005) offer some empirical evidence of this in the pharmaceutical market.

Rice, and Alecxih 1995). The NAIC designs required all Medigap plans to cover benefits viewed as important but unavailable in the market because of adverse selection incentives (for example, home health and prevention services). The result was a more stable market that offered a set of benefits that had eroded in the unregulated market (Rice and Thomas 1992).

We propose a similar process leading to formulation of a set of seven to nine standardized PDPs. A panel conceived for that purpose would include a mix of individuals representing various segments of the industry (PBMs, health insurers, drug manufacturers, and pharmacies) as well as consumer interests. The NAIC panel that designed the Medigap plans consisted of six individuals representing insurers and six representing consumers; a similar composition would be sensible in this case. The standardized plans would include the existing one specified in the MMA plus three to four new plan types that would be actuarially equivalent and another three to four enhanced plans. We further propose that within the groups of actuarially equivalent plans and extended plans, there be one or two different tiered formulary structures, one or two different deductible arrangements, and one or two different approaches to doughnut hole coverage (for example, coverage of generics only and coverage of generics and branded drugs).[12]

We believe that the resulting six to eight additional plans would allow for meaningful variation in plan offerings with respect to deductibles, cost sharing, and mail order coverage among both the actuarially equivalent and the enhanced plans. In addition, research on effectiveness of choice in 401(k) retirement plans indicates that employers offering ten or fewer plan choices have significantly higher employee participation than those offering more choices (Sethi-Iyengar, Huberman, and Jiang 2004).

Finally, standardization of plans would allow the CMS to address another problem. Recall that a substantial proportion of people who did not enroll in Part D would have been eligible for a low-income subsidy, and that many who did enroll likely selected a plan that did not offer the lowest expected out-of-pocket costs. The behavioral economics literature suggests that modifying default options for benefit plans can increase enrollment and improve choices (Thaler and Sunstein 2003), and the use of specific default options to improve decisionmaking in Part D and in Medicare generally has been suggested by McFadden (2006) and Frank (2007),

---

12. It has been argued that plan standardization might dampen innovation in benefit design. To address this issue, one standardized plan in each category might be designated an "experimental" plan, which a firm could propose and try out for a limited period. That firm could add no other new plan unless one was eliminated.

respectively. Under this approach, all new Medicare beneficiaries would be automatically assigned to a designated default plan from among the new standardized plans; the default plan would be an actuarial equivalent of the standardized plan offering the "best" insurance features for the average enrollee. New Medicare beneficiaries not interested in participating in Part D would have to actively opt out.

This approach is not so dissimilar from the automatic enrollment option now used with the Medicaid-eligible population and other identified low-income individuals. We expect that it would result in expanded enrollment among beneficiaries eligible for the low-income Part D subsidy, and perhaps among others as well. In addition, it would require participants to make an active choice to enroll in a plan that lacked attractive financial properties for the average beneficiary. The approach thus preserves freedom of choice but reduces some negative outcomes associated with human inertia or confusion.

COMPETITION FOR REGIONAL PLAN CONTRACTS. We also propose reorienting the nature of PDP competition, from competition for enrollees toward competition for contracts to offer the standardized plans. Although standardization of plans would simplify choices and allow enrollees to make more effective price-coverage comparisons, important dimensions of the care management process would remain that cannot be contracted for in advance. Formulary designs and utilization management arrangements cannot be completely regulated; hence important selection incentives will persist.[13]

One striking example of selection behavior was an enhanced benefit plan offered by Humana in 2006 that provided coverage for brand name drugs during the doughnut hole phase. Humana was the only insurer to offer such coverage (several companies offered plans with coverage of generic drugs in the doughnut hole). Beneficiaries who expected to spend amounts sufficient to reach the doughnut hole and who were on a brand name drug naturally gravitated to the Humana plan. As a result, Humana suffered substantial losses on the plan, their stock price fell, and in 2007 they did not offer such a plan. But in 2007 Sierra Health Plan offered a plan that covered brand name drugs in the doughnut hole, and, like Humana in 2006, it was the only insurer offering such coverage. History repeated itself; beneficiaries spending large amounts using brand name

---

13. The reduced number of generous enhanced plans in the second year of Part D suggests selection behavior is at work in this market.

drugs moved from the Humana plan to the Sierra plan. Like Humana, Sierra suffered losses and complained that Humana had telephoned its highest-cost customers to recommend they purchase from Sierra instead. Humana responded that they were only passing along information to their customers about a plan that might better suit their needs.

Therefore we propose that in each of the thirty-four regions, one contract be awarded to a single insurer for a limited period, on the basis of price, quality, and formulary design criteria. The duration of the contract should be set so that the threat of contract loss with poor performance is credible. Each insurer seeking a region's contract would submit a separate bid for each of the seven to nine standardized plans, along with formulary design plans.[14] The price bids would be evaluated by considering, for each bidder, the weighted average of its bid prices across the standardized plans. The initial weights could be based on current enrollments in the major classes of existing plans. Under standard models of competition, however, it is welfare improving for low-option plans to subsidize high-option plans (Rothschild and Stiglitz 1976). Some incentive in this direction could be given if the evaluation overweighted enrollment in high-option or generous plans, thereby giving bidders an incentive to increase enrollment in these plans. But even if this wrinkle were not adopted, one insurer would be granted all of an entire region's PDP business for the contract period, which would considerably reduce its adverse selection incentives. This proposal has the further advantage of maintaining considerable choice of plan types and creating incentives for price competition in premiums.[15]

This model of purchasing more closely resembles the PBM procurement methods of private health insurance plans than does the existing Part D structure, and in fact it is very similar to that of an employer that carves out its drug benefit. Given competition across thirty-four separate regions, there is little chance that a single plan sponsor would become dominant nationally; thus competition would be preserved for future contract negotiations. Maintaining robust future competition for contracts could be further strengthened by limiting the aggregate national Medicare PDP market share of a single firm, for example, to 30 percent.

---

14. The formulary design criteria might include an assessment of whether a majority (or a supermajority) of potential enrollees would find the drugs they take on the proposed formulary.

15. For a general discussion of the advantages of competition for contracts in prescription drugs, see Huskamp and others (2000).

This proposal would require the CMS to run thirty-four regional procurement processes for the standardized plans, similar to those it now runs for intermediaries and carriers to administer Parts A and B. Although that would be a new administrative task for the agency, it is not clear whether it would, on net, add to its administrative load. Recall that the agency in 2006 reviewed and processed premium bids, formulary design plans, and a utilization management arrangement for 1,429 plans, and for 1,875 in 2007. Nonetheless, selecting the "winner" of a franchise-like competition in each region could be more administratively demanding than simply approving plans, and therefore our proposal could result in higher administrative costs.

Competition for exclusive contracts for all Part D participants within a region may not be achievable politically. In that case, a useful fallback would be to employ it only for the institutionalized population. Before Part D, nursing homes mainly dealt with their state's Medicaid plan and their long-term care pharmacy provider when obtaining drugs for their residents. They now must deal with many plans with different formularies, potentially causing confusion and adding administrative cost. We see little advantage to this situation and believe there is an even stronger case to implement competition for contracts in the nursing home setting than for Part D generally. Whether the competition takes place at the level of the individual nursing home, the nursing home chain, or the region is a question we leave open. Given the needs of nursing home residents and their relatively high prevalence of cognitive impairment, a single plan might also be required to have a more open formulary than Part D plans presently offer. This would effectively set up an entirely separate drug benefit for the institutionalized, but we believe there is much to be said for this approach.

Filling the Doughnut Hole

As described above, the coverage gap or doughnut hole in the standard Part D plan requires enrollees to pay 100 percent of the cost of their prescription drugs for total expenditures between $2,400 and $5,451. This leaves beneficiaries exposed to out-of-pocket costs totaling $3,850 before the catastrophic coverage provisions kick in. As already noted, standardized and actuarially equivalent PDPs are prohibited from increasing the size of the deductible to reduce the size of the doughnut hole.

Projections for 2006 indicated that in that year about 4 million Part D participants, or 25 percent of the total, would incur expenses in the

doughnut hole not covered by low-income subsidies.[16] Among these participants, average out-of-pocket spending was estimated to be approximately $2,530.[17] Roughly 70 percent of those who encountered the dough-
nut hole would not cross the catastrophic coverage threshold, and only
about one-third were expected to incur spending of $1,500 or less.

The doughnut hole awkwardly balances concerns about the cost of providing a truly valuable drug insurance benefit with the desire to extend that
benefit to as many recipients as possible. But relaxing the prohibition on
increasing the deductible can increase the welfare of recipients even while
adhering to existing budget rules. In other words, benefit designs that are
actuarially equivalent to the current standardized design can offer typical
Medicare beneficiaries better protection (McFadden 2006).

We propose shifting this trade-off—between offering more insurance
protection and providing more people with benefits—in the direction of
the former. This could be accomplished by relaxing restrictions on the ability of PDPs to offer actuarially equivalent plans that provide greater coverage in the doughnut hole. In particular, allowing larger deductibles in combination with more complete doughnut hole coverage would move plans
toward more valuable protection against larger losses and away from less
valuable up-front, first-dollar protection. This is exactly what basic insurance principles imply.

A second measure would be to mandate coverage of generic medications in the doughnut hole, the most common form of coverage offered by
enhanced benefit plans. Generic drugs are widely prescribed: about 50 percent of all prescriptions are for generics, and the rate is even higher among
the lower-income elderly.[18]

Few precise data are available on the cost of extending coverage of
generic drugs in the doughnut hole, but the incremental premiums required

16. See Juliette Cubanski and Patricia Neuman, "Status Report on Medicare Part D
Enrollment in 2006: Analysis of Plan-Specific Market Share and Coverage," *Health Affairs*,
web exclusive, November 21, 2006 (content.healthaffairs.org/webexclusives/index.dtl?year=
2006).

This estimate is based on the assumption that 15 percent of enrollees in Part D are in
enhanced plans that offer coverage in the doughnut hole; it excludes the low-income group
from the denominator since there is no doughnut hole for them.

17. PricewaterhouseCoopers, "Significance of the Coverage Gap under Medicare Part D,"
June 8, 2006 (www.medicaretoday.org/clientuploads/directory/toolbox_resources/HLC
Brief60806.pdf).

18. Cindy P. Thomas, and others, "Impact of Health Plan Design and Management on
Retirees' Prescription Drug Use and Spending 2001," *Health Affairs*, web exclusive, December 4, 2002 (content.healthaffairs.org/cgi/content/abstract/hlthaff.w2.408).

for such coverage appear quite modest (MedPAC 2006, table 7-8). Existing data suggest that such coverage would increase premiums by at most $21 a month for existing plans (Hoadley and others 2006).[19] But the benefits of such a reform could be great. Coverage in the doughnut hole may result in higher rates of adherence to treatment regimens among those with chronic disease. This, in turn, might mean financial savings for Parts A and B of Medicare through averted spending, not to mention better health outcomes for beneficiaries (Hsu and others 2006; Fendrick and others 2001).

Improving the Cost Effectiveness of Purchasing

One of the promises of Part D was that elderly Americans could benefit from the bargaining power of larger and more sophisticated purchasers. PDPs were expected to build on advances in purchasing practices observed in the private sector, and in particular the emergence of the PBM industry and its use of formularies. Thus the design of Part D represents a substantial departure from the take-it-or-leave-it pricing that Medicare uses for all other medical goods and services, as well as from the principle that services from all providers should be available for almost the same price.[20] The private sector approach to purchasing, however, works best when there is robust competition. That requires the existence of multiple therapeutic substitutes so that PDPs can obtain a favorable price by steering greater numbers of people to buy one drug rather than another in response to favorable price offers from manufacturers (Frank 2001; Newhouse 2004).

EXPECTATIONS FOR DRUG PRICES UNDER PART D. The design features of Part D were based on some specific conceptions of price dynamics in the market for prescription drugs (CBO 2002). In general, the expectation was that most prices would fall with the introduction of Part D, or at least not increase notably. These expectations relied on notions of how prices are set for various segments of the market.

Medicare recipients who had no drug coverage before 2006 generally paid the highest prices in the market because they purchased through retail pharmacies. Retail pharmacies have little bargaining power over the prices they pay for branded prescription drugs, reflecting their inability to implement a formulary that would enable them to shift purchases

---

19. This is an upper bound because of selection against existing plans by those expecting to spend in the doughnut hole and use generic drugs.

20. The 20 percent coinsurance in Part B creates modest differences among prices charged by physicians for the minority of beneficiaries who pay the coinsurance, and some further difference is created by the minority of physicians who do not accept assignment.

among competing products (Frank 2001). These recipients were therefore expected to benefit from lower drug prices under Part D because their drug purchasing would now be made through PDPs, which do have formularies and other means of steering demand toward products on which price concessions are offered. For this group, the shift in purchasing arrangements has the effect of making demand for individual products in most drug classes more price responsive.

In contrast, drug prices for those dually eligible for Medicare and Medicaid were expected to rise, but only modestly (CBO 2002, chapter 3), because of two offsetting factors. Before 2006 dually eligible individuals had drugs purchased for them through Medicaid's "best price" rebate system, described above (Scott-Morton 1997). Under Part D, these beneficiaries were automatically shifted to PDPs, which operate under special rules. If they negotiate prices below Medicaid's "best price," these prices are not counted under the best price system. This creates a bargaining advantage for PDPs over other private plans, which should lower prices. At the same time, however, the enactment of Part D meant that demand for prescription drugs generally was sure to increase, creating upward pressure on prices because of the market power of most branded drugs. The expected net effect was a modest price rise.

Finally, unique drugs that offer important clinical advantages to elderly users pose a challenge to the Part D approach to prices because of the monopoly power such drugs enjoy (Newhouse 2004). Nevertheless, it was expected that this issue would have little overall effect on prices paid, for three reasons. First, it was thought that unique drugs were few in number and would remain unique for only a short time (CBO 2002; Newhouse, Seiguer, and Frank 2007). Second, the substantial cost sharing within the doughnut hole under Part D was expected to serve as a constraint on pricing. Third, the private sector would purchase a substantial volume of such medications and would use more powerful negotiating tools to contain costs (CBO 2002).

WHAT ACTUALLY HAPPENED. As we describe below, prices actually paid by Medicare in the initial phases of the Part D program appear to differ from expectations in some respects. In particular, for the 29 percent of Part D enrollees who are dually eligible for Medicare and Medicaid, the shift from the "best price" model of purchasing to the commercial PDP models seems to have resulted in significant rather than modest increases in the prices paid to manufacturers. Why this may be so is a matter of speculation. Because the market for PDPs is currently quite fragmented, because PDPs receive substantial subsidies from Medicare, and because they face only small levels of financial risk, their ability to shift between similar drugs and bargain hard with manufacturers may be more limited than previously expected. As a result, the impact on Part D spending may be greater than was anticipated.

The prices obtained by PDPs for drugs that had been heavily used by dually eligible beneficiaries can offer some insight into the ability of PDPs to get the best private prices. Unfortunately, these prices cannot be directly compared because both Medicaid and PDP prices are confidential. Some information about the pricing environment, however, can be gleaned from examining the public financial statements of drug manufacturers during the first six months of 2006, which assess the impact on manufacturer revenue from shifting the dually eligible from Medicaid to PDP pricing arrangements.

We reviewed manufacturers' Form 10-Q filings with the Securities and Exchange Commission and looked for commentary or data on drugs that are heavily used by dually eligible Part D participants. One class of such drugs is antipsychotic medications, 70 percent of which were purchased by Medicaid before January 2006. AstraZeneca (maker of Seroquel), Bristol-Meyers Squibb (Abilify), Eli Lilly (Zyprexa), and Pfizer (Geodon) all noted favorable (for them) changes in prices resulting from the shift of large numbers of users of antipsychotic medications from Medicaid to Part D. For example, Bristol-Meyers Squibb stated that the shift in patient enrollment to Part D had a positive impact on the company's bottom line, which was partly offset by a negative impact in the managed care side of the business. Similarly, Lilly noted an increase in effective net selling prices for Zyprexa, partly due to the transition of certain low-income patients from Medicaid to Medicare. Finally, Pfizer pointed to a more general impact of the price gains from the payment shift: the company saw a $325 million increase in revenue from this source for the first six months of 2006 compared with the same period in 2005, or approximately an 8 percent increase in net revenue. A clear inference from these figures is that PDPs are not obtaining prices that approximate the best price in the private market. Manufacturers have realized significant gains simply from the change in responsibility for purchasing from Medicaid to Medicare.[21]

---

21. It is highly unlikely that the higher prices represent a move to an efficient price because for several drug classes that relied largely on sales to Medicaid, such as the antipsychotic class described in the text, there were high rates of entry of new drugs. We infer that expected revenue at Medicaid prices was sufficient to encourage research and development for new products in those classes.

In the case of unique drugs, as already noted, PDPs are potentially in a weak bargaining position because they have limited ability to redirect demand away from the unique product. Moreover, in the Medicare context, there will surely be strong political pressure not to allow PDPs to leave unique—and presumably superior—products off the formulary. Thus the threat of exclusion because of a high price is unlikely to be credible, and because of the formulary regulations—which are set on clinical, not economic, considerations—it may even be precluded. The incentive for a PDP to bargain hard with the manufacturer is further blunted by the fact that the government is responsible for 80 percent of an individual beneficiary's drug costs above $5,450, and the beneficiary for 5 percent. Thus the PDP faces only a 15 percent liability for beneficiaries in this range of spending. (In the case of specialty drugs, which frequently carry high prices, the consumer is responsible for 25 percent of the cost and the government 75 percent.)

Because the insurer shares the cost with others, the manufacturer of a unique drug, especially one heavily used by the elderly, may be able to set a price that is much higher than that of a monopolist selling to an uninsured market and still sell the same quantity.

In other words, the manufacturer's market power comes not only from the patent(s) it holds but also from the patient's insurance coverage: outside the doughnut hole, the patient faces little or no incremental cost from a higher price. As a result, consumer demand for drugs is markedly less responsive to the monopolist's price than it would be in a market of uninsured consumers, the usual case outside of health care. The combination of a lack of competing drugs and insurance that covers a high percentage of the patient's cost effectively puts the patent system on steroids.

How important are unique drugs in the marketplace? New drugs with important therapeutic advantages are regularly introduced into existing therapeutic classes, and some new products result in the creation of new classes. Significant market power can arise in either case. In other work we have identified drugs that were the first to appear in their class. Between 1970 and 2000, the number of such drugs averaged about 3.5 a year (Newhouse, Seiguer, and Frank 2007). Recently that number has dropped markedly: only five drugs brought to market were first in their class in the entire period between 2000 and 2004—just one a year on average. In recent years, drugs that were first in their class have remained in that position for about three years.

Identifying drugs that offer unique therapeutic advantages within an existing class is more difficult than identifying first-in-class drugs. But we can point to some recent examples, including Forteo, which treats osteoporosis, and Plavix, which treats heart disease. In addition, some drugs maintain a dominant position in sales to elderly Americans despite having therapeutic competitors. Such drugs include Norvasc, an antihypertensive, Xalatan for glaucoma, and Toprol for heart disease. Thus we believe the enhanced market power for manufacturers created by Part D has the potential to create a distributional imbalance, offering substantially greater economic rents to the manufacturers of some drugs than would be observed in an uninsured market. Any such rents, of course, further aggravate the parlous future financial health of Medicare.

There are indications that prices have responded in the anticipated fashion. Some of the most significant price changes during the first half of 2006 reported by manufacturers of branded prescription drugs occurred in drugs that were relatively unique and had high shares of elderly buyers. Examples include Plavix, Forteo, and Evista (another drug used in preventing osteoporosis).

To explore such price effects more systematically, we compared two subgroups of drugs selected from the top fifty best-selling prescription drugs in the United States. The first subgroup consisted of the ten branded drugs with elderly usage shares of 55 percent or greater; the second consisted of the ten branded drugs with elderly shares of less than 35 percent. None of the drugs in either group had generic equivalents on the market. Figure 6-2 plots price indexes for the two groups. These indexes moved at identical rates during the year before passage of the MMA but began to diverge during 2004 and to move further apart around January 2006, when Part D was implemented.[22] By June 2006 there was a 6 percentage point difference between the indexes, favoring the drugs with high elderly shares. We attribute this divergence to the changes in Part D for the dually eligible population and enhanced pricing power for unique drugs.[23] The extent to which these prices will continue to diverge in the future, of course, remains unknown.

OBTAINING BETTER PRICES WHILE PRESERVING INNOVATION INCENTIVES. Any proposal to alter approaches to setting prescription drug prices must

22. By contrast, Berndt and others (1998) found that during the early 1990s price indexes for drugs used by the elderly did not differ significantly from those for drugs used by others.

23. Other sources offer consistent observations. For example, the American Association of Retired Persons (AARP) reports larger increases in the average cost of treating chronic conditions of the elderly between 2005 and 2006 than in any of the previous five years. AARP, "Prices of Brand-Name Drugs Continue to Rise Faster than Inflation," *Rx Watch Drug Report*, September 2006.

Figure 6-2. Price Indexes for Drugs Used by the Elderly and the Nonelderly[a]

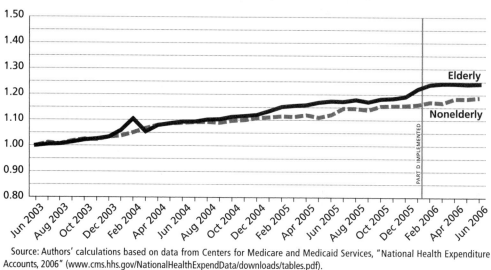

Source: Authors' calculations based on data from Centers for Medicare and Medicaid Services, "National Health Expenditure Accounts, 2006" (www.cms.hhs.gov/NationalHealthExpendData/downloads/tables.pdf).
a. Price indexes are Laspeyres indexes.

recognize the threat posed to research and development (R&D) incentives and to the industry's ability to attract capital if prices are set "too low." Pharmaceutical R&D has generated enormous economic value in recent decades (Murphy and Topel 2003). Moreover, many important diseases, including Alzheimer's disease and many cancers, still have little effective therapy, so further R&D will likely prove valuable. Thus the key trade-off sets the risk of reduced R&D incentives against bestowing additional economic rents on the pharmaceutical industry and creating greater stress on an already troubled federal budget.

Recent assessments of the evidence suggest that the pharmaceutical industry's profitability does modestly exceed that of the Fortune 500, even after one adjusts for intangible capital and differences in risk (CBO 2006a, chapter 6). Furthermore, analyses of incentives in prescription drug markets that stem from patents and insurance subsidies suggest that incentives for excessive innovation exist (Garber, Jones, and Romer 2006). Since Part D represents an important expansion of insurance subsidies in pharmaceuticals, any preexisting incentive to overinvest in R&D is an important consideration.

On the other hand, unique, clinically important drugs are by definition exactly those from which society benefits most by offering large rewards to drug manufacturers. Focusing cost control efforts on these drugs may impose particular risks on precisely the R&D that should be most encouraged.

As a first step toward establishing a better balance between control of Medicare spending and protection of R&D incentives, we propose that manufacturers be required to sell drugs to PDPs for use by dually eligible beneficiaries at prices that approximate the previous Medicaid prices. This would serve to restore the balance to its pre-January 2006 level, a set of prices that appeared acceptable to all parties. The impact on Medicare spending would likely be significant, given that the dually eligible account for an even larger share of Part D drug purchases than their 29 percent share of the Medicare population. There should be little additional administrative cost. PDPs would report their purchases on behalf of dually eligible enrollees, and the manufacturer would provide a corresponding rebate to the federal government, much as rebates are now provided to Medicaid.

We believe that it is premature to conclude that enough unique drugs exist today to create a meaningful budget problem. Therefore we propose that the prices of such products be carefully monitored and that government be prepared to intervene if such a problem arises. If it does, we propose that the government put in place temporary administered prices for unique drugs. The goal would be to establish a price for Medicare Part D that preserves R&D incentives, recognizes the potential health benefits of new products, and limits the economic rents paid by the Medicare program. The establishment of this price could be accomplished through a system of binding arbitration or via rate setting as in the rest of Medicare. Under either case, the government would develop a price proposal.

The first step in developing a temporary price proposal for a given unique drug would be to project the per unit price that would allow the manufacturer to recoup its R&D costs given the expected volume of sales in the United States and abroad, and the average cost of developing a new drug with the specific attributes in question. We recognize that most drug R&D involves joint costs across a number of products, making any such calculation inherently arbitrary to some degree. We propose, for simplicity's sake, that the joint costs be allocated according to the ex ante volumes of sales across the drugs in question. The aim of using the expected costs and domestic and foreign sales volumes in the calculation is to arrive at a base price that supports an expected break-even point plus some margin. This was the method used by the Office of Technology Assessment (1990) to recommend a Medicare reimbursement level for erythropoietin (an anti-anemia drug). Using such a price preserves incentives for manufacturers to conduct both R&D and product launch activities efficiently.

We would then propose an adjustment to the base price to take account of the drug's unique health benefits. This would be done by calculating the improvement in cost per quality-adjusted life year offered by the new drug over the average existing treatment and adjusting the price accordingly. The adjustment would thus reflect any increase in willingness to pay for the drug's clinical advantages, such as would be expected to occur in a well-functioning market (Lu and Comanor 1998; Reinhardt 2004). The aim here is to offer greater economic rewards for new products that offer more important benefits. This would serve to give greater weight to R&D that promises relatively better health outcomes per dollar.

The temporary administered price would remain in place until the entry of two additional drugs offering meaningful therapeutic competition to the drug in question (Bresnahan and Reiss 1991). At that point, price determination would revert to the market.

Regulation of price and insurance coverage of new prescription drugs in other nations uses some similar concepts in establishing prices for new drugs. In Australia the government negotiates prices based on evidence on cost-effectiveness (also measured in cost per quality-adjusted life year), prices of alternative products, cost information provided by manufacturers, prescription volume, overseas prices, and the importance of the selling firm to the Australian economy. The relative cost-effectiveness of the new drug is used to establish a price premium for any therapeutic advantages it offers (Birkett, Mitchell, and McManus 2001).

U.K. pharmaceutical regulation establishes a rate-of-return corridor for firms across the whole of their business in the United Kingdom. An important feature is that new products are exempted for their first five years on the market. The accounting is complicated, in part because of the aforementioned problem of allocating joint costs of R&D. This approach seems impractical for application in the limited context that we propose since our proposal would apply primarily to newer products, and the rate of return at the firm level will by and large not be relevant. Because the proposal focuses on pricing above the expected break-even point, the new products will contribute positively to the rate of return of the innovating firm.

Finally, a variety of commentators have suggested that Medicare set prescription drug prices based on those currently obtained by the Department of Veterans Affairs (VA). We think this approach would be unwise, for four main reasons. First, the VA not only purchases drugs but also dispenses them from centralized pharmacies staffed by VA employees. This is dramatically different from relying on retail pharmacists to distribute prescription drugs as is done under Medicare and Medicaid. For this reason alone, Medicare beneficiaries would not have prescription drugs available to them at VA prices. Yet the costs of dispensing are typically left out of price comparisons in the literature. In addition, the VA uses closed formularies for a number of drug classes and exerts a great deal of management control over its employee physicians to ensure adherence to formulary rules. Such procedures would likely not be acceptable to either Medicare beneficiaries or their physicians.

Third, Medicare is a very large purchaser, acquiring prescription drugs for over 40 million people. Extending the VA discount beyond purchases for veterans would certainly change the economics of the bargaining between the VA and prescription drug manufacturers, such that prices to the VA would rise. Such a change in bargaining occurred following the implementation of Medicaid's "best price" scheme, resulting in higher prices to the VA and the Department of Defense. In short, if Medicare based prescription drug prices on VA prices, the VA would no longer be able to negotiate prices as advantageous as those it obtains today. Finally, even if VA prices could be negotiated for Medicare, those prices might be so low as to threaten incentives for R&D, thereby compromising the future supply of innovative new drugs.

Consolidating Drug Benefits under Part D

Medicare Part B has long covered drugs that are usually administered by clinical personnel as opposed to those taken orally or otherwise self-administered. In 2004 Part B drugs accounted for over $10 billion in Medicare outlays (MedPAC 2006), and spending on these drugs has risen at a rapid rate, roughly doubling between 2001 and 2004. Cost sharing for Part B drugs differs from that under Part D: beneficiaries simply pay 20 percent of the cost of the drug, with no upper limit. Some beneficiaries have additional retiree health insurance that covers this cost, as does Medicaid.

Medicare currently reimburses purchasers of Part B drugs, typically physicians, 106 percent of the national average sales price (ASP). Especially for drugs with a high Medicare share, this is an open invitation for the manufacturer to name a high price since that price can simply be passed through to the government, except for any copayment. Not only does the manufacturer reap the direct benefit of a high price, but the physician also has a greater incentive to dispense a high-priced drug, despite the availability of cheaper therapeutic competitors, because the physician earns 6 percent of the ASP (Jacobson and others 2006).[24]

We propose abolishing the distinction between Part B and Part D drugs and instead covering all drugs under Part D.[25] To minimize transition issues, existing cost sharing for Part B drugs could be grandfathered for a period of time. ASP reimbursement, however, would end: PDPs would negotiate a price with manufacturers for current Part B drugs as they do now for Part D drugs. We propose, however, that whatever is done with cost sharing for these drugs be done on a budget-neutral basis, that is, projected federal spending for Part B drugs would simply be added to the federal subsidy for Part D.

Consolidating all drug coverage under Part D would end the confusing and arcane regulations surrounding what qualifies a drug for coverage under Part B rather than Part D. It would also end the incentive a manufacturer now has, when a choice of delivery mechanism arises for a new drug, to consider whether Part B or Part D coverage would maximize reimbursement. Clearly reimbursement should not influence that choice. More generally, the distinction between Part B and Part D drugs does not meet the "how-would-you-explain-it-to-your-mother" test. It is simply an anachronism from the time when Medicare did not cover most drugs but did cover some under Part B.[26]

Conclusions

Medicare Part D has benefited millions of elderly Americans who before 2006 either had no insurance coverage against prescription drug spending or had very limited and expensive coverage. It has been especially helpful to lower-income elderly Americans (those below 135 percent of the poverty line) who did not qualify for Medicaid because under Part D they receive generous subsidies to aid in purchasing prescription drugs.

24. This discussion ignores the incentive of the physician to account for the burden to the patient from any coinsurance.

25. For the institutionalized population, a small step in this direction has been taken by shifting some drugs previously covered by Part B to Part D, namely, those defined as "incident to" a physician's service. See Centers for Medicare and Medicaid Services, "Medicare Parts B/D Coverage Issues" (www.cms.hhs.gov/Pharmacy/Downloads/partsbdcoverageissues.pdf).

26. If Part B drugs are moved to Part D, PDPs would have to demonstrate adequate capabilities to contract with those dispensing the drugs and to deliver them appropriately (many need refrigeration). However, major PDPs now handle such drugs for their commercial enrollees, sometimes through a separate specialty pharmacy entity, so we do not see this requirement as an important barrier to entry.

Elements of the design of Part D, however, force it to underachieve. It presents Medicare beneficiaries with an overwhelming array of choices and a large variety of different and complicated benefit structures. The result for many is confusion, which discourages some from enrolling at all and leads others to choose plans that do not best serve their financial interests. The program allows a great deal of leeway for PDPs to design their own formularies and adopt a variety of drug utilization management strategies. Although this freedom should lead to better tailoring of plans, it can also enable PDPs to engage in risk selection.

The design of the program also shifted several million dually eligible people away from Medicaid's drug purchasing arrangements, resulting in a substantial price increase for the drugs they use. Furthermore, by prohibiting the government from direct involvement in price negotiations for Part D drugs, the law has put manufacturers in a position where, for drugs with few or no therapeutic competitors, they can more or less name their price. This is a potentially untenable situation given the serious looming pressures on the federal budget. Finally, the legislation preserved a confusing and anachronistic distinction between Part B and Part D drugs.

We therefore propose a set of seven measures that should improve consumers' ability to choose among PDPs, reorient price competition to discourage adverse selection by plan sponsors, improve the insurance features of the basic coverage, and change the basis of price negotiations for an important subset of prescription drugs so as to lower their cost. The specific policy changes we propose are as follows:

—Standardize benefit designs to between seven and nine plan types. This would simplify plan offerings while still maintaining meaningful choice in coverage.

—Reorient competition for enrollees to competition for exclusive contracts to sell the standardized plans in each of the designated thirty-four regions. This would remove the strong incentives for sponsors to compete for low-risk enrollees. If this is not acceptable politically, then at a minimum, implement such a reform for the nursing home population.

—Assign every new Medicare enrollee a Part D plan as a default option. This should correct some errors now often made by consumers, especially failure to enroll or to enroll in the "best" plan because of misunderstanding, while still preserving free choice for those who want to exercise such choice.

—Alter the regulations governing the basic benefit so that actuarially equivalent plans can offer coverage in the doughnut hole. This could be done by allowing PDPs to offer plans with higher deductibles together with doughnut hole coverage, or by extending the basic benefit so that generic drugs are covered in the doughnut hole.

—Return prices paid on behalf of dually eligible beneficiaries to levels that approximate pre-Part D Medicaid prices. This would serve to balance concerns over the growing Medicare budget with the legitimate need of the pharmaceutical industry to recoup its R&D costs.

—Monitor the prices of therapeutically unique drugs and develop a standby method of establishing temporary administered prices for such drugs. Such prices would be used only if unique drugs create important budget strains and would be removed when sufficient competition emerged to make price competition likely.

—Move all drugs now covered under Part B to Part D, on a budget-neutral basis. If desired, existing Part B cost sharing could be grandfathered for some period.

Taken together, these measures would preserve the basic principles of private provision, price competition, and enrollee choice upon which Part D was founded while redressing imbalances that we believe have placed consumers and public budgets at an excessive disadvantage. These measures also focus explicitly on the need to balance responsible pricing and the burdens placed on the federal budget with the critical need to maintain incentives for innovation that will result in new and better prescription drugs for future generations of Americans.

References

Berndt, Ernst R., and others. 1998. "Is Drug Price Inflation Different for the Elderly? An Empirical Analysis of Prescription Drugs." In *Frontiers in Health Policy Research*, vol. 1, edited by Alan M. Garber. MIT Press.

Birkett, Donald J., Andrew S. Mitchell, and Peter McManus. 2001. "A Cost Effectiveness Approach to Drug Subsidy and Pricing in Australia." *Health Affairs* 20, no. 3: 104–14.

Borschow, Jason. 2007. "Filling in the Gaps: Examining the Effects of the Medicare Prescription Drug Benefit Design on Beneficiary Drug Utilization." Harvard University, Department of Economics.

Bresnahan, Timothy F., and Peter C. Reiss. 1991. "Entry and Competition in Concentrated Markets." *Journal of Political Economy* 99, no. 5: 977–1009.

Camerer, Colin F. 2000. "Prospect Theory in the Wild." In *Choices, Values and Frames*, edited by D. Kahneman and A. Tversky, pp. 288–300. New York: Cambridge University Press.

Congressional Budget Office (CBO). 2002. *Issues in Designing a Prescription Drug Benefit*.

———. 2004. *A Detailed Description of CBO's Cost Estimate for the Medicare Prescription Drug Benefit.*

———. 2006a. *Research and Development in the Pharmaceutical Industry.*

———. 2006b. *The Budget and Economic Outlook.*

———. 2007. *The Budget and Economic Outlook: Fiscal Years 2008–2017.*

Fendrick, A. Mark, and others. 2001. "A Benefit-Based Copay for Prescription Drugs: Patient Contribution Based on Total Benefits, Not Drug Acquisition Cost." *American Journal of Managed Care* 7, no. 9: 861–67.

Fox, Peter D., Thomas Rice, and Lisa Alecxih. 1995. "Medigap Legislation for Health Care Reform." *Journal of Health Politics, Policy and Law* 20, no. 1: 31–48.

Frank, Richard G. 2001. "Prescription Drug Prices: Why Do Some Pay More than Others Do?" *Health Affairs* 20, no. 2: 115–28.

———. 2007. "Behavioral Economics and Health Economics." In *Behavioral Economics and Its Applications,* edited by Peter Diamond and Hannu Vartiainen, pp. 195–221. Princeton University Press.

Garber, Alan M., Charles I. Jones, and Paul M. Romer. 2006. "Insurance and Incentives for Medical Innovation." Working Paper 12080. Cambridge, Mass.: National Bureau of Economic Research (March).

Hoadley, Jack, and others. 2006. "Benefit Design and Formularies of Medicare Drug Plans: A Comparison of 2006 and 2007 Offerings. A First Look." Report 7589. Menlo Park, Calif.: Kaiser Family Foundation.

Holtz-Eakin, Douglas. 2003. "Prescription Drug Coverage and Medicare's Fiscal Challenges." Testimony before the Committee on Ways and Means, House of Representatives. Congressional Budget Office (April 9).

Hsu, John T., others. 2006. "Medicare Drug Benefit Caps: Unintended Consequences." *New England Journal of Medicine* 354, no. 22: 2349–59.

Huskamp, Haiden A., and others. 2000. "The Medicare Prescription Drug Benefit: How Will the Game Be Played?" *Health Affairs* 19, no. 2: 8–23.

Jacobson, Mireille, and others. 2006. "Does Reimbursement Influence Chemotherapy Treatment for Cancer Patients?" *Health Affairs* 24, no. 2: 437–43.

Kaiser Family Foundation. 2006a. "Medicare Prescription Drug Coverage among Medicare Beneficiaries: Data Update." Publication 7453. Menlo Park, Calif.

———. 2006b. "Seniors and the Medicare Prescription Drug Benefit: Chartpack." Publication 7604. Menlo Park, Calif.

———. 2007. "The Medicare Prescription Drug Benefit: Fact Sheet." Publication 7044-06. Menlo Park, Calif.

Lu, John Z., and William Comanor. 1998. "Strategic Pricing of New Pharmaceuticals." *Review of Economics and Statistics* 80, no. 1: 108–18.

McFadden, Daniel. 2006. "Free Markets and Fettered Consumers." *American Economic Review* 96, no. 1: 5–29.

Medicare Payment Advisory Commission (MedPAC). 2006. *Report to Congress: Increasing the Value of Medicare.*

Murphy, Kevin M., and Robert Topel. 2003. "The Value of Medical Research." In *Measuring the Gains from Medical Research: An Economic Approach,* edited by K. Murphy and R Topel, pp. 41–73. University of Chicago Press.

Newhouse, Joseph P. 2004. "How Much Should Medicare Pay for Drugs?" *Health Affairs* 23, no. 1: 89–102.

Newhouse, Joseph P., Erica Seiguer, and Richard G. Frank. 2007. "Was the Medicare Drug Bill a Giveaway to the Pharmaceutical Industry?" *Inquiry* 44, no. 1: 15–25.

Office of Technology Assessment. 1990. *Recombinant Erythropoietin: Payment Options for Medicare.* OTA-H-451. Government Printing Office.

Pauly, Mark V., and Yuhui Zeng. 2004. "Adverse Selection and the Challenges to Stand Alone Prescription Drug Insurance." In *Frontiers in Health Policy Research,* vol. 7, edited by David Cutler and A. M. Garber, pp. 55–74. MIT Press.

Reiffen, David, and Michael Ward. 2005. "Generic Drug Industry Dynamics." *Review of Economics and Statistics* 87, no. 1: 37–49.

Reinhardt, Uwe E. 2004. "An Information Infrastructure for the Pharmaceutical Market." *Health Affairs* 23, no. 1: 107–12.

Rice, Thomas, and Kathleen Thomas. 1992. "Evaluating the New Medigap Standardization Regulations." *Health Affairs* 11, no. 1: 194–207.

Rothschild, Michael, and Joseph Stiglitz. 1976. "Equilibrium in Competitive Insurance Markets: An Essay on the Economics of Imperfect Information." *Quarterly Journal of Economics* 90, no. 4: 629–50.

Scott-Morton, Fiona. 1997. "The Strategic Response by Pharmaceutical Firms to the Medicaid Most Favored Customer Rules." *RAND Journal of Economics* 28, no. 2: 269–90.

Sethi-Iyengar, Sheena, Gur Huberman, and Wei Jiang. 2004. "How Much Choice Is Too Much? Contributions to 401(k) Retirement Plans." In *Pension Design and Structure: New Lessons from Behavioral Finance,* edited by O. S. Mitchell and S. Utkus, pp. 83–95. Oxford, U.K.: Oxford University Press.

Simon, Kosali I., and Claudio Lucarelli. 2006. "What Drove First Year Premiums in Stand Alone Drug Plans?" Working Paper 12595. Cambridge, Mass.: National Bureau of Economic Research (October).

Thaler, Richard H. 1999. "Mental Accounting Matters." *Journal of Behavioral Decision Making* 12, no. 3: 183–206.

Thaler, Richard H., and Cass R. Sunstein. 2003. "Libertarian Paternalism." *American Economic Review* 93, no. 2: 175–79.

U.S. Government Accountability Office. 2006. *Medicare Part D: Prescription Drug Plan Sponsor Call Center Responses Were Prompt, but Not Consistently Accurate and Complete.* GAO-06-710.

Wrobel, Marian V., and others. 2003. "Predictability of Prescription Drug Expenditures for Medicare Beneficiaries." *Health Care Financing Review* 25, no. 2: 37–46.

The Promise of Progressive Cost Consciousness in Health Care Reform

7

JASON FURMAN

In 1965 the average American received $995 worth of medical care (in today's dollars).[1] Nearly half of this amount, $483, was paid out of pocket for deductibles, copayments, coinsurance, or for services and supplies not covered by insurance. Third parties, usually private insurance companies, paid the other half. In the decades that followed, health care was transformed as increased use of health care services, together with expensive new technologies and drugs, increased spending per capita to an estimated $6,640 in 2006. Yet even as national health care spending increased nearly sevenfold, the amount that consumers paid out of pocket did not even double, rising to just $837 in 2006. Most of the remainder of health spending, now over 87 percent of the total, was covered by

The author wishes to thank Henry Aaron, Gary Claxton, David Cutler, Douglas Elmendorf, Judy Feder, Eve Gerber, Robert Greenstein, Jonathan Gruber, Arnold Kling, Leighton Ku, Larry Levitt, Suzanne Nora-Johnson, Edwin Park, Meeghan Prunty-Edelstein, Robert Reischauer, Jonathan Skinner, and Lawrence Summers for helpful comments. Rebecca Kahane, Ariel Levin, and Iris Lin provided helpful research assistance.

1. Calculated using data from the Centers for Medicare and Medicaid Services (CMS), "National Health Expenditure Accounts, NHE Historical and Projections, 1965–2016," 2007 (www.cms.hhs.gov/NationalHealthExpendData/03_NationalHealthAccountsProjected.asp#TopOfPage), and from the Bureau of Economic Analysis (BEA), "Gross Domestic Product: Fourth Quarter 2006 (Preliminary)" (www.bea.gov/newsreleases/national/gdp/2007/gdp406p.htm). All inflation adjustments use the price index for personal consumption expenditures.

insurance. Public insurers (mainly Medicare and Medicaid) and private insurers each pick up roughly half the tab. In other words, by 2006 the average household was directly paying for about one-eighth of its health care, down from one-half in 1965. Today the average American pays a smaller fraction of health expenses out of pocket than the average resident pays in other high-income countries, all of which have universal insurance.

On balance, the transformation of health care financing has been a positive development. Insurance coverage has been extended to many who before were without it, and the benefits that the typical American receives are far more comprehensive than they used to be. This expansion of health insurance has led to better access to health care, and this in turn has contributed to longer life expectancy and improvements in the quality of life—benefits that far exceed their cost (Cutler, Rosen, and Vijan 2006; Hall and Jones 2007; Murphy and Topel 2006). Although too many people remain exposed to too much health-related financial risk, insurance does protect most households from the enormous variation in health care expenditure to which the vagaries of illness would otherwise subject them. According to the 2004 Medical Expenditure Panel Survey (MEPS), though most families spend a substantial amount on health care, the spending is relatively predictable, with 96 percent of nonelderly households in the middle-income quintile spending less than 10 percent of their income on out-of-pocket payments for health care.[2]

At the same time, Americans are frustrated with health care. They worry about the overall level of expenditures that are putting a strain on family and government budgets. They worry about the high and rising number of uninsured. And they worry about whether they are getting enough value for their money. Some have touted high-deductible health plans associated with health savings accounts (HSAs) or new tax deductions for health expenses (Cogan, Hubbard, and Kessler 2005) as the magic bullet solution to all these problems. Not only are these approaches not magic bullets, but

---

2. See U.S. Department of Health and Human Services, Agency for Healthcare Research and Quality, "Medical Expenditure Panel Survey (MEPS)," 2004 (www.meps.ahrq.gov/mepsweb). The MEPS has been conducted annually since 1996 (data are available up to 2004). Its predecessor surveys were the National Medical Care Expenditure Survey (NMCES), conducted in 1977 (National Center for Health Services Research 1977), and the National Medical Expenditure Survey (NMES), conducted in 1987 (Agency for Healthcare Research and Quality 1987). Although the 1977 and 1987 surveys are not fully comparable to the MEPS, comparisons with the Bureau of Labor Statistics' Consumer Expenditure Survey and the CMS National Health Expenditure data indicate that the data are reasonably consistent for our purposes. Nonelderly households are defined as those headed by someone under the age of sixty-five.

they also create significant and unnecessary problems, including exposing low- and moderate-income families to too many financial risks, possible worse health outcomes, and costly and regressive tax cuts that in many cases have little to do with health care (see Collins 2006; Furman 2006b).

Although proponents of HSAs have the wrong prescription, their diagnosis captures one important problem with our current health system. What we need is a different approach to encourage cost consciousness in a progressive manner that links the level of cost sharing to income and attempts to use cost sharing to improve systemwide incentives for more effective care. This approach has the potential to be not just more equitable but also more economically efficient than the HSA approach. Moreover, even those who would rather not see any more cost sharing should recognize that greater cost sharing is likely to be part of the health system in the future. That makes it all the more important to help ensure that this cost sharing is designed in an efficient and fair manner that reduces major risks, promotes better health, and makes health insurance more affordable.

The effect of increased insulation from prices on household decisions about health care has several downsides. First, because few people are confronted with the full price of their care, more care tends to be purchased: physicians order more tests, procedures, and drugs for their patients; hospitals invest in more expensive equipment and have the incentive to use it more; and medical innovation favors exotic technologies over technologies that lower costs. The insulation from the full cost of health care has been responsible for anywhere from 10 to 50 percent of the large increase in health expenditures as a share of the economy in recent decades (Manning and others 1987; Finkelstein 2007). Households may be insulated from paying for health care out of pocket, but they cannot be shielded from paying the full cost through other means, including premium payments, forgone wages to cover the cost of employer premium contributions, and higher taxes to pay for public programs (see, for example, Gruber 1994). These add up, putting an increasing strain on family budgets and reducing real wage growth. For example, in 2006 a typical working-age family of four had an income of about $97,000 (including employer benefits) and paid $16,153, directly and indirectly, for health care—17 percent of that family's total income (see box 7-1).

Second, the decline in out-of-pocket spending relative to total health spending is one of the major factors in the disturbing increase in the number of uninsured, from 14 percent of the nonelderly population in 1987 to 17 percent of that group in 2005 (DeNavas-Walt, Proctor, and Smith 2007). When out-of-pocket costs are lower, premiums must necessarily be

Box 7-1. How Does a Typical Family Pay for Health Care?

Health care expenditures	Dollars[a]	Percent of income
Employee contribution to premium	2,973	3
Out-of-pocket expenses for cost sharing	1,643	2
Employer contribution to premium	8,508	9
Income and Medicare payroll taxes	3,029	3
Total	16,153	17

Source: Author's estimates using data from a variety of sources including U.S. Census Bureau and U.S. Bureau of Labor Statistics, "Current Population Survey, March 2005" (www.census.gov/cps); Bureau of Labor Statistics, "Employer Costs for Employee Compensation" (www.bls.gov/news.release/ecec.toc.htm); U.S. Department of Health and Human Services, Agency for Healthcare Research and Quality, "Medical Expenditure Panel Survey (MEPS)," 2004 (www.meps.ahrq.gov/mepsweb); and Kaiser (2006).

a. All data are updated to 2006 dollars.

higher. This is partly a matter of simple accounting—costs not borne out of pocket must be covered—and partly a matter of the economic incentives just described: people will use more health care when the price they pay for one more doctor's visit or one more prescription is low. The result is that health insurance itself is increasingly expensive, leaving more households unwilling or unable to pay for coverage. Moreover, many households are underinsured and left facing substantial financial risks: 22 percent of workers are in plans that have no out-of-pocket maximum, exposing them to potentially unlimited risks (Kaiser Family Foundation, the Health Research and Educational Trust, and the Center for Studying Health System Change [Kaiser] 2006).[3] Even families with good insurance plans face the risk and associated anxiety of losing that coverage.

Finally, the transformation in health care financing can lead to worse health outcomes. Those who go without insurance receive less than half as much health care as the insured, resulting in poorer health outcomes for them, including an estimated 18,000 premature deaths annually (Committee on the Consequences of Uninsurance 2003).[4] Those who do have insurance spend more but do not necessarily get better outcomes. On average, health spending is enormously beneficial, with benefits that far outweigh its costs. At the margin, however, the effectiveness of health spending varies greatly. Much of it is ineffective or even harmful. The

3. Some of these workers are in HMOs and thus face little cost sharing, making the absence of an out-of-pocket limit irrelevant to the risks they face.

4. See also Jack Hadley, and John Holahan, "Covering the Uninsured: How Much Would It Cost?" *Health Affairs*, web exclusive, June 4, 2003 (content.healthaffairs.org/cgi/content/full/hlthaff.w3.250v1/DC1).

RAND Health Insurance Experiment (see below) found that a large majority of people who did not face any cost sharing received 40 percent more health care without any better outcomes than those who had cost sharing, in part because the extra spending went to procedures that were barely useful or even harmful. A number of studies have identified large disparities in the intensity of treatments for Medicare patients in different parts of the United States, without any commensurate difference in outcomes.[5] One survey noted that "for patients with hip fractures, colorectal cancer, or myocardial infarction, more conservative practice patterns are associated with better survival" (Fisher 2003, p. 1665). Direct studies of medical procedures have found that a large fraction—often totaling one-third of all such procedures—are either inappropriate or of equivocal value (McGlynn 1998). At the same time, some health spending is clearly underutilized, in particular some preventive care and well-proven drugs to control chronic conditions such as hypertension, diabetes, and depression. At a systemwide level, there are few incentives to help direct people toward health care that is extremely important and underutilized and away from other seemingly more common areas where care is marginal or even harmful. Moreover, some of the techniques to get more out of health spending—for example, health maintenance organizations (HMOs)—have been increasingly unpopular, in part because the supply-side constraints, whereby insurance companies deny treatments or give health providers an incentive not to offer care, are not consistent with the demand-side incentives, which offer patients the prospect of free care, with no cost sharing, for any approved procedures.

Helping consumers become more cost conscious about their health care choices, if and *only* if it is done correctly, has the potential to generate progress in three areas. First, greater cost consciousness can bring down health insurance premiums. The progressive cost-sharing plan presented in this chapter would lower total health spending by 13 to 30 percent and premiums by 22 to 34 percent. Employers' savings on premium contributions would be passed on to workers in the form of more rapidly rising wages, alleviating some of the squeeze that families face. Second, greater cost consciousness can reduce the number of uninsured, both directly by making premiums more affordable and indirectly as part of a broader health care reform that uses some of these savings to ensure affordable universal coverage. Moreover, exposing families to smaller expenses can help

---

5. See, for example, John E. Wennberg, Elliot S. Fisher, and Jonathan S. Skinner, "Geography and the Debate over Medicare Reform," *Health Affairs,* web exclusive, February 13, 2002 (content.healthaffairs.org/cgi/reprint/hlthaff.w2.96v1.pdf).

shield them from larger expenses. In the progressive cost-sharing plan, at least 23 percent of people would see their out-of-pocket expenses fall, particularly families with lower incomes or larger out-of-pocket expenses in the current system. Finally, by more appropriately aligning medical evidence and system-side incentives facing both patients and providers, more cost-effective insurance may also promote health. All told, increasing cost sharing for most everyday health care expenditures, such as low-yielding medical tests, while reducing the income share that households have to pay for catastrophic care, can lower total health care spending, improve health outcomes, and ultimately reduce the financial risks faced by families.

One key to implementing cost consciousness correctly is to provide more protection to households with low and moderate incomes, and more direct exposure to price signals for higher-income households. Reforms along these lines have been proposed by people across the ideological spectrum, from conservative economist Martin Feldstein (1971) to single-payer health insurance supporter Thomas Rice (Rice and Thorpe 1993).[6] Ideally, this could be accomplished simply by linking the degree of cost sharing in insurance plans to income—for example capping out-of-pocket payments at 7.5 percent of income for middle-class families. If income-linked out-of-pocket payments prove too difficult to institute, lower-income households could instead be compensated for the extra risks associated with greater cost sharing by providing them with lower premiums—or even tax credits or transfers—to help them meet their out-of-pocket payments.

Also worth considering is some form of "smart" cost sharing that would exempt health treatments that have proven benefits but are currently underutilized, such as preventive care, statins for people with high cholesterol, or beta-blockers to manage cardiac arrhythmias.[7] Covered participants would pay nothing or a reduced amount out of pocket for these favored treatments. Not only would this lower the relative price of these treatments to users, but it would also send a strong signal about the types of care that are proven to be valuable and effective from a wellness point of view. Moreover, extra cost sharing would ideally be combined with some form of compensation for those with chronic conditions. The current limitations of our knowledge about both medical effectiveness and how the utilization of different types of treatments responds to prices, however, limit what we could accomplish with smart cost sharing today.

6. See also Feldstein and Gruber (1995); Seidman (1980).
7. See Lambrew, chapter 8 in this volume.

Nevertheless, the potential payoffs to getting it right are high enough that further research and experimentation would be very beneficial.

If done incorrectly, however, greater cost sharing could be counter-productive. Consider the high-deductible insurance plans associated with the HSAs established under the Medicare Prescription Drug, Improvement, and Modernization Act of 2003.[8] These plans have a fixed deductible, which averages $4,000 for a family plan, and returns on savings within the associated accounts accumulate tax free (Kaiser 2006). Each family has the same deductible regardless of its income, leading to a substantial risk for lower-income families who may not be able to afford the $4,000 deductible while only negligibly changing the health care spending incentives facing high-income families. Moreover, not only do low-income families get the extra risk, but they also get little benefit from the tax-free accounts because they are in low tax brackets. In contrast, high-income families are able to bear the risk *and* get tax breaks that are larger for people in higher tax brackets. In some cases, these tax breaks actually increase the bias of the tax code toward greater health care spending, potentially increasing total health expenditures (Furman 2006b; Remler and Glied 2006). Moreover, under current law, HSAs also lack any mechanism to insure people with chronic conditions. Finally, the integration of cost sharing into health care reform needs to be mindful of the ever-present potential for adverse selection: healthier people tend to opt into plans with more cost sharing to take advantage of the lower premiums, leading insurers to try to differentiate between the healthy and the less healthy and to exclude the latter from coverage or price it out of their reach. But because today's HSAs were introduced in the absence of comprehensive health reform that addresses this problem, they actually increased the risk of adverse selection, splintering insurance pools.

Cost consciousness is not a magic bullet. It is also important to combine cost sharing, which is a demand-side approach to improving the cost effectiveness of care, with supply-side measures that lead to better decisions about which care is offered and to whom. These include familiar managed care techniques such as reviewing the use of health care and giving suppliers the incentive to offer appropriate care through supply-side cost sharing (whereby suppliers share some of the costs of treatment) and pay for performance (which rewards doctors and hospitals for achieving measurable benchmarks). Instead of demand- and supply-side measures being viewed as alternatives, however, they can and should be viewed as complements

8. P.L. 108-173.

(Newhouse 2004). Indeed, one reason for the backlash against managed care in the past decade may have been the disconnect between the demand and supply sides: consumers were promised essentially free care, only to be told when they came to seek care that they could not have it. If demand-side incentives and supply-side constraints can be made to work together, the result might be a more effective and more sustainable health care environment than Americans experienced under the rigid managed care techniques associated with HMOs that became increasingly unpopular in the late 1990s.

Enhanced cost consciousness is not without its downsides. It presents a trade-off: health insurance can become more affordable, and individuals can face a smaller risk of personal financial catastrophe—but only if all of us accept an increased financial risk over a range of possible spending that falls far short of catastrophic levels. Because risk is an inherently random process, this means that some individuals will inevitably end up better off and others worse off. If the alternative to greater cost consciousness were free care with no constraints at a low premium, the choice would be easy, but this is not the choice we face. In a world of limited resources, where illness strikes unpredictably and all health care must ultimately be paid for by individuals, trade-offs are unavoidable. The goal of increased cost consciousness is to help put individuals in the position to make their own decisions about these trade-offs.

Cost consciousness can and should be a critical component—together with pooling mechanisms to ensure that everyone has an affordable insurance option—of any viable plan to achieve such universal coverage. Even single-payer health insurance needs a way to decide what care to provide or to withhold in order to keep costs from rising uncontrollably. Most countries with single-payer plans do this in part through cost sharing. In fact, as detailed below, the United States has a lower overall rate of cost sharing than the average member country of the Organization for Economic Cooperation and Development (OECD). Health reforms at the U.S. state level that include an individual mandate, like the Massachusetts plan, face the challenge of designing a pooling option that is affordable enough for middle-class families who receive little or no subsidies. Income-related cost sharing is one way to meet this challenge.

Raising cost consciousness is not a cure-all. The challenges facing the nation's health care system are so large that no single change can hope to solve all of them. Better information technology, improved disease management, more effective prevention, and strategies to address the mounting public health challenges, such as the obesity epidemic, will all be important in ensuring that we get the maximum benefit from our health dollars. In some areas, particularly managing chronic illnesses, we should spend more, not less.

But none of these reforms, by themselves, address the difficult problem of deciding when and how to say no to expensive care of marginal benefit (Aaron, Schwartz, and Cox 2005). In an economy that relies on the ability of individuals to make sound decisions in their own interest, and in a society that is concerned about individual outcomes, exposing individuals to the price of health care through greater cost sharing, in a manner consistent with their ability to pay, is a sensible approach. Although not necessarily popular, neither are the alternatives: having insurance companies or the government make these decisions or allowing health expenditures to grow without bound.

This chapter argues for serious consideration of a greater role for cost consciousness in health care reform, provides evidence of the potential of this greater role, and also warns about the dangers of approaches such as current law HSAs. However, this chapter does not propose a single, specific reform design because any cost-sharing measure or set of measures chosen should be part of a broader health system reform that provides universal insurance, and the form of cost sharing will depend on the shape of that system. Instead, the goal is to provide guidance for how cost sharing could be included in broader reforms.

The next section reviews recent trends in cost sharing, and in particular the long-term decline in cost sharing relative to total health care spending. The subsequent section examines the evidence on cost sharing and finds that it has the potential to dramatically lower costs with no adverse effect on health or financial security—provided that cost sharing is related to income. This is followed by an analysis of the impact of alternative forms of cost sharing, focusing on income-related out-of-pocket limits. The focus then briefly shifts to some important related issues, including the potential for "smart," evidence-based cost sharing and how best to insure the chronically ill. The penultimate section sketches some ways to implement income-related cost sharing, or versions of it, and the final section summarizes the role of progressive cost sharing in health care system reform.

Trends in Cost Sharing

In the United States today, the majority of families face relatively little cost sharing, either as a fraction of their income or as a fraction of their total health care expenditure. As noted in the introduction, the costs borne directly by those with insurance have diminished as a share of total health care spending, and that share is lower than the average for other OECD economies.

It is worth emphasizing at the outset that *cost sharing* as used here is limited strictly to out-of-pocket payments by the health care consumer, either for services not covered by insurance or for the portion of covered services that, under the insurance contract, the insured must pay for through deductibles, copayments, and the like. The definition does not include premium payments, including those paid directly by the insured individual and indirectly through the lower wages that reflect the employer's contribution. There are three reasons for this focus. First, this analysis is concerned with factors that affect the amount of health care a person receives, measured both in terms of total spending and in terms of its impact on that person's health. Here the most relevant factor is how much a person has to spend for health care actually consumed, not how much she or he pays for insurance. Second, some conventional estimates of the individual's share of health care spending are flawed because they do not reflect the fact that even insured individuals ultimately bear the full burden of that spending, either through direct expenditure on premiums or through out-of-pocket payments, lower wages, or higher taxes. Finally, the emphasis here is on the risks associated with health care spending. Variable out-of-pocket payments, which can range from nothing to hundreds of thousands of dollars, represent a risk. A known premium, whether paid by an employer or by the individual, does not. This is not to say that rising premiums, or more generally a rising share of income devoted to purchasing health insurance, are not also cause for concern, but this concern is part of what motivates the focus on out-of-pocket payments and their role in health care spending in the first place.

This section begins with an analysis of aggregate data that capture broad trends in both public and private insurance. Then it uses data at the individual level to focus on changes in cost sharing for the privately insured. Finally, it puts cost sharing in the United States in a comparative international perspective.

Cost Sharing Has Declined Relative to Total Health Care Spending, Both in the Aggregate . . .

The Centers for Medicare and Medicaid Services (CMS) compiles the National Health Expenditure Accounts, the official federal government statistics on aggregate health care spending. These statistics document the transformation of health care and its financing since 1960. At that time, before the invention of so many of the lifesaving but costly technologies

Figure 7-1. Aggregate Cost-Sharing Rate, 1960–2006

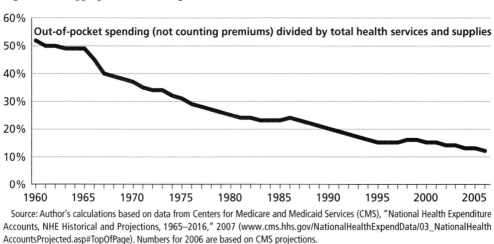

Source: Author's calculations based on data from Centers for Medicare and Medicaid Services (CMS), "National Health Expenditure Accounts, NHE Historical and Projections, 1965–2016," 2007 (www.cms.hhs.gov/NationalHealthExpendData/03_NationalHealth AccountsProjected.asp#TopOfPage). Numbers for 2006 are based on CMS projections.

and drugs that have come to define modern medicine, the average health care consumer spent much less on health care than today. But Americans have been paying a smaller and smaller fraction of their health care costs out of pocket, from just over 50 percent in 1965 to just under 13 percent in 2006. Figure 7-1 shows a clear and continuous downward trend in the share of health care spending spent directly on health care goods and services. The trend has slowed, however, although not actually stabilized, in the past decade.

Again, this is not to say that individuals do not have to pay for their rising health care spending. Ultimately, individuals pay 100 percent of the cost of health care, and this cost is rising as a share of income. But much (and today the majority) of that expenditure comes in the form of rising contributions to health insurance premiums, lower wages (to compensate employers for their contribution to employees' health insurance), and higher taxes to pay for public health care programs.[9] What figure 7-1 illustrates is

9. The total share of health spending that comes directly from individuals—the sum of individual premium payments and out-of-pocket health payments—has fallen nearly continuously, from 61 percent in 1960 to 28 percent in 1980 to an estimated 22 percent in 2006. The share of health care paid by employers rose from 16 percent in 1960 to 30 percent in 1980 and has stayed at roughly that level ever since. Over the same period, the share of health care paid by government has risen nearly continuously, from 23 percent in 1960 to an estimated 47 percent in 2006. These statistics are not very meaningful, however, because they do not reflect who ultimately pays the cost of health care.

Figure 7-2. Out-of-Pocket Health Spending as Percent of Income and Consumption, 1960–2006

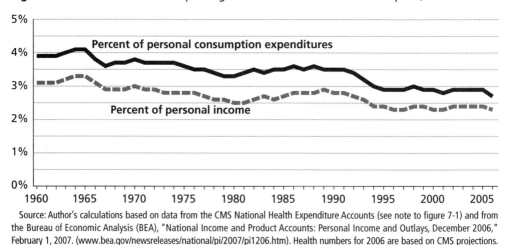

Source: Author's calculations based on data from the CMS National Health Expenditure Accounts (see note to figure 7-1) and from the Bureau of Economic Analysis (BEA), "National Income and Product Accounts: Personal Income and Outlays, December 2006," February 1, 2007. (www.bea.gov/newsreleases/national/pi/2007/pi1206.htm). Health numbers for 2006 are based on CMS projections.

a transformation in how individuals pay for health care spending—paying a substantially larger fraction in advance and less in real time as they use the health goods and services. As noted earlier, this is what matters for the financial risk that families face and their level of spending.

Out-of-pocket payments are declining, not only as a share of total health care spending but also as a share of aggregate personal income and of personal consumption expenditure, as figure 7-2 shows. The former is especially remarkable because total health services and supplies tripled as a share of income from 1960 through 2006.

Together these aggregate figures tell a crude but broadly accurate story about the expansion of insurance over the past forty years. In part, they capture trends in cost sharing for private insurance policies, but they also capture the broader expansion in public and private insurance coverage. Several factors explain why out-of-pocket health care expenditure per capita has remained relatively flat relative to income and total consumption, even as it has declined dramatically relative to total health care spending.

First, public insurance coverage has expanded. The aggregate cost-sharing rate dropped by nearly 10 percentage points after the introduction of Medicare and Medicaid in 1965, and these programs have continued to bring this rate down. The percentage of the nonelderly enrolled in Medicaid increased from 8 percent in 1987 to 13 percent in 2005

(DeNavas-Walt, Proctor, and Smith 2007). Since Medicaid has historically had virtually no cost sharing, this shift toward Medicaid has reduced aggregate cost sharing—although this is now changing somewhat because many states have begun to increase cost sharing in their Medicaid programs, particularly after the Deficit Reduction Act of 2005 (Artiga and O'Malley 2005; Ku and Wachino 2005). In addition, the implementation of a new prescription drug benefit in Medicare starting in 2006 has transferred much of the burden of paying for drugs from individual patients to private insurance companies and the government, further reducing the cost-sharing rate.[10]

Second, although cutbacks by insurance companies garner plenty of press and popular attention, the long-term trend in private insurance has been toward providing increasingly comprehensive benefits. Health insurance originated as a system for covering hospitalization. As late as the 1960s and 1970s, many insurance plans offered only limited coverage for ambulatory services: in 1977 individuals paid for 52 percent of the cost of doctors' visits out of pocket. In recent decades, virtually all insurance companies have added coverage for these services, with the portion of doctors' visits paid out of pocket falling to 14 percent in 2004.[11] At the same time, coverage for prescription drugs has gone from rare to nearly universal, while coverage for mental health care, chiropractic services, dental care, and other health services is also becoming more common. The large majority of these expenses used to be covered entirely out of pocket.

Finally, cost sharing has evolved within private insurance itself, mainly in tandem with the shift toward managed care. The share of Americans with employer-sponsored insurance enrolled in some form of managed care rose from 2 percent in 1979 to 97 percent in 2006 (Henderson 2005; Kaiser 2006). The shift to managed care—HMOs, preferred provider organizations, and the like—put people into plans that offered lower cost sharing than most fee-for-service plans. In fact, 88 percent of workers covered by HMOs pay no deductible at all (Kaiser 2006), in exchange for more supply-side constraints on participants' use of care services. Other data from the 1990s reflect this trend toward managed care: although deductibles rose for most types of care, the shift toward plans with lower

10. A notable exception is that some low-income families who are eligible for both Medicaid and the Medicare prescription drug benefit have seen their costs go up. See Frank and Newhouse, chapter 6 in this volume.

11. Based on data from the NMCES (National Center for Health Services Research 1977) and the U.S. Department of Health and Human Services, Agency for Healthcare Research and Quality, "Medical Expenditure Panel Survey (MEPS)," 2004 (www.meps.ahrq.gov/mepsweb).

deductibles (usually managed-care plans) meant that the average worker faced a falling deductible.

The high-water mark of this transformation was in 1996, when 31 percent of workers were enrolled in HMOs, which represented a doubling in the HMO share in just eight years. The share of workers enrolled in HMOs fell back to 20 percent in 2006 as many people rebelled against the supply-side constraints on their care (Kaiser 2006). As a result, health expenditures rose rapidly and insurance companies started to return to cost sharing in order to control expenses.

Ultimately, the goal of insurance is to balance two competing interests. On the one hand, individuals want to be protected against the risks associated with fluctuations in their income or expenditure needs. On the other hand, this protection leads to "moral hazard," resulting in more total spending and thus crowding out money for other priorities. The key is to strike a balance between these two competing needs. The fact that out-of-pocket payments have fallen relative to income and consumption implies that the risk associated with health expenditures has declined over time.[12] The reduction in the aggregate cost-sharing rate implies that the distortions associated with moral hazard have grown over time. To the degree that we were striking the right balance at any point in the past, this broad analysis suggests that we are no longer striking the right balance today.

. . . and among Those with Private Insurance

The decline in cost sharing in the aggregate captures a broad set of phenomena, including the spread of insurance and changes in the nature of insurance. This subsection uses data at the individual level (that is, microdata) to focus on the evolving pattern of health expenditure for the nonelderly, including a focus on those with private insurance.

Table 7-1 demonstrates that cost sharing, again relative to total health care expenditure, is also declining among the nonelderly with private insurance. (Results for those with public insurance or for the elderly, which are not shown, are very similar.) The first row shows that the trend for this subgroup is similar to the aggregate trend depicted in figure 7-1.[13] The second row shows that the level of cost sharing is higher for the median

12. Strictly speaking, this is true if utility functions exhibit constant relative risk aversion, which is commonly assumed to be the case.

13. These estimates are slightly higher, in part because they use a different data set and in part because of differences in coverage. For example, the aggregate cost-sharing data include in the denominator the administrative costs incurred by insurance companies whereas these are not reflected in the microdata.

Table 7-1. Measures of Coinsurance for Nonelderly Households with
Private Insurance[a]

Units as indicated

Measures	1977	1987	1996	2004
Aggregate cost-sharing rate (percent)	35	27	20	19
Median household cost-sharing rate (percent)	59	41	29	25
85th percentile household cost-sharing rate (percent)	100	90	67	56
Median out-of-pocket spending/income (percent)	1.3	1.2	0.9	1.3
85th percentile out-of-pocket spending/income (percent)	5.0	4.5	3.5	4.3
Mean out-of-pocket spending (2006 dollars)	1,183	1,323	1,046	1,451
Median out-of-pocket spending (2006 dollars)	674	699	571	828
Standard deviation of out-of-pocket spending (2006 dollars)	1,718	2,870	1,568	2,038

Source: Calculations using the NMCES (National Center for Health Services Research 1977), the NMES (Agency for Healthcare Research and Quality 1987), and the 1996 and 2004 MEPS (U.S. Department of Health and Human Services, Agency for Healthcare Research and Quality, "Medical Expenditure Panel Survey [MEPS]" [www.meps.ahrq.gov/mepsweb]).
a. Private insurance is limited to families who are privately insured throughout the year.

household than for households in the aggregate, largely because the average rate is driven down by very large payments by insurers for a minority of families. But the downward trend in cost sharing—relative to health expenditures—is even more pronounced for the median household, perhaps because of the increasing importance of extreme expenditures that are covered by insurance. Because health expenditure is thus skewed across families, the third row reports the cost-sharing rate at the eighty-fifth percentile. This, too, displays a similar trend.

The fourth and fifth rows of the table show that out-of-pocket health spending has been relatively stable as a share of income for median households and has declined a little for households with especially high medical expenses.[14]

The table's bottom three rows report actual (inflation-adjusted) dollar values for out-of-pocket spending at the mean and the median of the distribution, as well as the standard deviation. What is noteworthy here is that

14. There are two reasons why the income ratio for the median household is flat and the ratio in figure 7-2 is falling. First, increased inequality means that aggregate income (shown in figure 7-2) is rising more quickly than median income (shown in table 7-1). Second, the definition of income used in figure 7-2 includes employer-provided benefits while the definition of income in table 7-1 excludes such benefits. Since these benefits have risen as a share of cash income, a broader measure of median out-of-pocket payments relative to income would be falling relative to the numbers shown in table 7-1.

Figure 7-3. Selected Consumer Expenditures, 1984 and 2005[a]

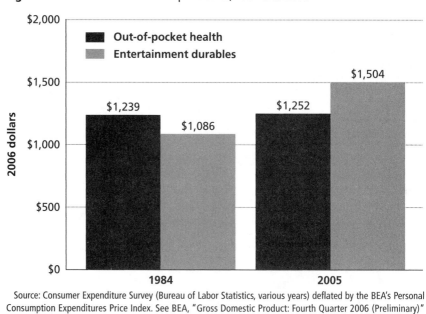

Source: Consumer Expenditure Survey (Bureau of Labor Statistics, various years) deflated by the BEA's Personal Consumption Expenditures Price Index. See BEA, "Gross Domestic Product: Fourth Quarter 2006 (Preliminary)" (www.bea.gov/newsreleases/national/gdp/2007/gdp406p.htm).
  a. Average for the middle quintile. "Entertainment durables" is "entertainment" minus "fees and admissions."

out-of-pocket health spending for both the average and the median family increased fairly little (relative to the surge in overall health spending) between 1977 and 2004.

While the long-term trends in cost sharing are falling relative to health expenditures and are stable relative to income or in real terms, cost sharing has increased substantially since 1996. As noted earlier, that year represents the peak of the experience with HMOs, most of which have little or no cost sharing. As HMO enrollment has declined—and managed care more broadly has become less strict—some of the cost sharing that characterized insurance in the 1970s and 1980s is returning.

Sometimes analysts treat any increase in the level of out-of-pocket spending as prima facie evidence of a problem, but spending on other goods and services has increased as well. Figure 7-3, which draws on yet another data set, the Consumer Expenditure Survey (Bureau of Labor Statistics, various years), shows that in 1984 consumers spent more on out-of-pocket health care expenses than on "entertainment durables" such

Table 7-2. Median Cost-Sharing Rates by Income Quintile for Nonelderly Families

Percent

Income quintile	1977	1987	1996	2004
Median cost-sharing rate				
Bottom	32	27	21	14
Second	57	46	32	24
Third	61	44	30	27
Fourth	56	38	31	27
Top	60	43	32	29
Median cost-sharing as a share of income				
Bottom	1.9	2.2	1.6	2.0
Second	1.7	1.7	1.3	1.3
Third	1.4	1.4	1.1	1.3
Fourth	1.1	1.1	0.9	1.1
Top	0.7	0.7	0.7	0.8

Source: See note to table 7-2.

as televisions and pets. By 2005 out-of-pocket health care spending was largely unchanged (in inflation-adjusted terms), but average spending on entertainment durables had increased by 40 percent.

Table 7-2 shows that cost sharing for households at each of several different levels of income has also declined over time.[15] In addition, it shows that, in any given year, rates of cost sharing for the top four income quintiles have been broadly similar, whereas the rate for the bottom quintile has been consistently lower. The pattern is reversed, however, when cost sharing is measured as a share of before-tax family income: families in the bottom quintile, on average, pay a much larger share of their income in out-of-pocket health care costs than do families at any other quintile.

Both the aggregate averages and the averages by income quintile obscure large differences in out-of-pocket spending from household to household. For two-thirds of nonelderly families in the middle-income quintile, this spending is less than 2 percent of their before-tax income (table 7-3). At the other end of the spectrum, an unlucky 4 percent of families devote

15. Note that family incomes are adjusted for family size by dividing by the square root of the number of people in the family, the procedure used by the Congressional Budget Office, among others. Table 7-2 includes all of the nonelderly, including both those in public and private health insurance. If the analysis is limited to the privately insured, it is still the case that the cost sharing has fallen in recent decades. However, for the privately insured, cost-sharing rates fall very slightly as income falls. The inclusion of Medicaid drives the much more rapid declines in cost-sharing rates shown in table 7-2.

Table 7-3. Distribution of Out-of-Pocket Expenses for Nonelderly Families, Middle-Income Quintile, 2004

Percent

Expenses as a percent of income	Distribution
Less than 2 percent	65
2–5 percent	23
5–10 percent	8
More than 10 percent	4
Total	100

Source: Author's calculations using 2004 MEPS data.

more than 10 percent of their before-tax income to out-of-pocket health care expenses. Figure 7-4 shows that the fraction of families facing these large expenses reached a low of 2 percent in 1999. Although that proportion has doubled since then, it remains at or below the levels that prevailed in the 1970s and 1980s. The recent increase is the result of three factors: incomes barely increased from 1999 to 2004, health expenditures increased at an even more rapid than normal rate during these years, and the rollback of HMOs and stricter managed care techniques gave rise to more cost sharing in order to control costs.

Cost-Sharing Rates Are Higher in Other Countries

Contrary to popular belief, the comprehensive national health insurance systems in many other industrial countries entail more, not less, cost sharing than the average U.S. family bears relative to total health spending. Data from the OECD show that the United States pays 13 percent of its national health care spending out of pocket—below the average of 17 percent in other high-income OECD countries (OECD 2006).[16] In effect, $1 of health care costs $0.13 in the United States and $0.17 in the rest of the high-income OECD nations (figure 7-5).

Nevertheless, the 13 percent figure might actually overstate cost sharing in this country. If the comparison were limited to the insured population in the United States—a more apples-to-apples comparison, given that the other industrial countries insure virtually their entire population—cost sharing in the United States would be lower.

16. The OECD average is weighted by population and excludes OECD countries with GDP per capita below $20,000 in 2005. Including these countries would raise the weighted average to 19 percent. The OECD data do not include an estimate for the United Kingdom.

Figure 7-4. Percentage of Families with Out-of-Pocket Payments above 10 Percent of Income, Middle-Income Quintile, Nonelderly, 1977–2004

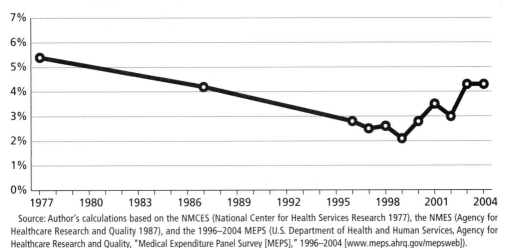

Source: Author's calculations based on the NMCES (National Center for Health Services Research 1977), the NMES (Agency for Healthcare Research and Quality 1987), and the 1996–2004 MEPS (U.S. Department of Health and Human Services, Agency for Healthcare Research and Quality, "Medical Expenditure Panel Survey [MEPS]," 1996–2004 [www.meps.ahrq.gov/mepsweb]).

Figure 7-5. Coinsurance Rates in High-Income OECD Countries, 2003

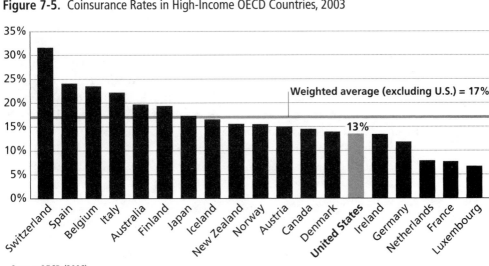

Source: OECD (2006).

What form does cost sharing take in the other industrial countries? Most impose cost sharing on pharmaceuticals and, to a lesser degree, on outpatient care. In France, for example, the public health system imposes a modest amount of cost sharing, but most people buy supplementary insurance that covers their copayments. It is also true, however, that health care systems in other industrial countries do not rely primarily on demand-side constraints but instead use global budget caps and rationing in ways that have no analogy in the United States.

Note that the United States has higher health spending overall, so out-of-pocket payments are substantially higher relative to income than they are in other countries. Therefore, the United States should optimally have a lower cost-sharing rate than other countries in order to keep the risk of health spending relative to income in check and even recognizing the extra distortion to incentives. The point of this comparison is not to explain the differences in spending between the United States and Europe or to argue that the United States should have the OECD average cost-sharing rate. Instead, these data are simply intended to emphasize that the debate over cost sharing should be separated from debates such as the one on the value of single-payer health insurance.

Evidence on the Impact of Cost Sharing

Cost sharing affects total health care spending, health outcomes, and the financial well-being of the households subjected to it; four decades of empirical research have accumulated considerable evidence on these impacts. Perhaps the best evidence comes from one of the most ambitious social science experiments ever conducted: the RAND Health Insurance Experiment, which lasted from 1974 through 1982 (Newhouse and the Insurance Experiment Group 1993, Manning and others 1987). This landmark research project randomly assigned 2,000 nonelderly families (comprising about 7,000 individuals) to fee-for-service plans with different levels of cost sharing. Researchers then collected detailed data on health expenditures and health status for the three to five years that these individuals were enrolled.[17]

The use of a random trial enabled the researchers to identify what effects were caused by the cost sharing itself. It avoided the difficult problem, inherent in research based on inferential statistical methods, of deter-

17. For a good summary of the RAND experiment and subsequent evidence, see Gruber (2006).

mining the direction of causality. For example, if higher cost sharing is found to be statistically associated with better health, is that because cost sharing leads to better health outcomes, or did the healthier people in the sample tend to choose plans that featured high cost sharing? The random assignment of families to different plans eliminates this ambiguity.

It is important to treat the RAND results cautiously and use a range of other evidence to confirm and update the conclusions. The RAND experiment, after all, was conducted twenty-five years ago, and some dramatic changes in health technologies (including the increased importance of prescription drugs and medical imaging) and the practice of insurance (most notably utilization review) have occurred since then. Moreover, the RAND experiment examined the behavioral effects of varying cost sharing assuming that the rest of the health system was unchanged. It has become increasingly clear that systemwide changes in cost sharing would have effects that go well beyond what could be captured in a randomized experiment.

Studies conducted since the RAND experiment have tended to confirm its finding of the effects of cost sharing on health expenditures and suggest that they might be even larger than the RAND study found. The studies have a less clear message of the effects of cost sharing on health outcomes, although they find that caution is warranted, at least for prescription drugs in certain populations.

Effects on Health-Care Spending

Several popular arguments cast doubts on whether cost sharing could have much of a real impact on health care spending. It is often argued that people will not respond to cost sharing because almost all health care is considered necessary: when their health is on the line, people will pay whatever their providers charge. As shown below, though, RAND and subsequent studies have found that people in fact do respond to higher out-of-pocket prices for health care: at the margin, people will consume less care if the cost is high.

Others argue that cost sharing will do little to hold down costs because total health care spending is driven by the exorbitant spending of a minority of consumers. In 2004, for example, 20 percent of nonelderly households were responsible for 70 percent of health care expenditures for the whole nonelderly population. People at that level of expenditure are generally well beyond the range where any significant cost sharing would apply.

This argument does identify an important limitation of cost sharing and the reason that cost sharing will never be a solo magic bullet solution to

Table 7-4. Utilization of Health Care in the RAND Health Insurance Experiment

Units as indicated

Plan	Probability of any medical use (percent)	Probability of inpatient use (percent)	Medical expenses per person (1991 dollars)
Free care	87	10.4	1,019
25 percent coinsurance	79	8.8	826
50 percent coinsurance	74	8.3	764
95 percent coinsurance	68	7.8	700

Source: Newhouse and the Insurance Experiment Group (1993, table 3.3, p. 44).

limiting care, and why supply-side constraints such as utilization review will likely always be a part of the health system. But in its simple form, the argument has two shortcomings. First, much of the expenditure of this high-spending 20 percent may still be subject to cost sharing. The typical high-deductible health plan includes cost sharing up to about $7,000 of total health care expenditures for individuals and $14,000 for families. In total, 86 percent of nonelderly households, representing 41 percent of total expenditures, fell under these limits and thus were subjected to cost sharing throughout the year. Moreover, even for people who eventually go above the limit, cost sharing might affect their initial spending, potentially affecting as much as the 61 percent of total health spending falling in the cost-sharing range. Second, all of these calculations are based on the assumption that the distribution of health care expenditure under current insurance practices would persist under a new system. In fact, the distribution is likely to change. For example, a patient with heart problems that are better treated by drugs but who undergoes marginally useful (or even harmful) surgery costing $100,000, who thus would appear to be unaffected by cost sharing at the margin, might not have undertaken the surgery at all in a world with more cost sharing.

The best way to evaluate the impact of cost sharing on health care is to look at the data, most notably RAND but also some recent studies. The RAND experiment assigned participants to one of five different plans, each with a different degree of cost sharing: completely free care (zero out-of-pocket spending), 25 percent coinsurance, 50 percent coinsurance, 95 percent coinsurance, or an outpatient deductible (table 7-4). The plans with coinsurance had an out-of-pocket maximum specified as the lower of a stated percentage of income (5, 10, or 15 percent) or a fixed dollar amount ($1,000—which is equivalent to $5,000 today if adjusted for per capita income growth, or $9,000 if adjusted for per capita health spending growth). Thus the 95 percent coinsurance plan effectively worked like a high-deductible plan. Individuals paid virtually the entire cost up to the maximum, at which point full coverage kicked in.

The right-hand column of table 7-4 shows how much participants in the free-care plan and in each of the different coinsurance plans spent on their health care. The findings clearly demonstrate that cost sharing can reduce health care spending. Participants paying 25 percent coinsurance spent 19 percent less than those with free care, and those subject to 95 percent coinsurance spent 15 percent less than those with 25 percent coinsurance. In total, going from free care to the plan with the highest deductible reduced spending by 31 percent. Using data for the whole sample, the RAND researchers estimated that the elasticity of health care spending to price was 0.22. In other words, a 10 percent increase in the price of health care would lead to a 2.2 percent reduction in use.

The RAND results further indicated that this reduction in spending was largely attributable to reduced contacts with health providers: people who went to a doctor or entered a hospital at all during the experimental period had relatively similar spending, regardless of the level of cost sharing. Also, consumption of each of the various types of health services—physician visits, hospital visits, emergency room visits, prescription drugs, and mental health care—responded similarly to a given percentage increase in price. Finally, there was no evidence that any of the spending reductions among those with high cost sharing were offset by more costly visits to the hospital later on, for example.

One important and much noted RAND group finding is that people in the experiment cut back just as much on care that was deemed necessary as they cut back on care that was deemed unnecessary, casting doubt on the proposition that people were making completely rational decisions. Presumably, people subject to cost sharing also cut back on care that was actually more harmful than beneficial, although the study did not explicitly identify such a category. The importance of this deviation from rationality is best measured by the impact of these changing patterns of use on health outcomes (covered in the next section). Moreover, an important policy question is how an individual's less-than-optimal choices compare to the less-than-optimal choices that would otherwise be made by insurance companies or by the government.

The RAND researchers also analyzed the price responsiveness of health care utilization by income. Their findings (table 7-5) corroborated those of other studies, which had found that even when care is free, families with

Table 7-5. Predicted Annual Use of Medical Services by Income Group

Units as indicated

Item	Bottom third of income group	Top third of income group
Probability of any use (percent)		
Free care	83	90
25 percent coinsurance	72	85
50 percent coinsurance	65	82
95 percent coinsurance	62	74
Average expenses (1991 dollars)[a]		
Free care	1,033	1,060
25 percent coinsurance	891	817
50 percent coinsurance	800	773
95 percent coinsurance	762	691

Source: Newhouse and the Health Insurance Experiment Group (1993, table 3.4, p. 46).
a. See table 7-4.

higher incomes are more likely to use medical services and to spend more money when they do use those services. As coinsurance rates rose, both higher- and lower-income participants became increasingly unlikely to use any medical services, and the gap between the two groups widened relative to free care. But in dollar terms, low-income households reduced their spending by less than high-income households, with families in the bottom third of the income distribution cutting their health spending by 26 percent when they switched from free care to 95 percent coinsurance, compared to a 35 percent reduction for families in the top third of the income distribution. As a result, lower-income families spent more, on average, on health care services than the higher-income families spent when both were enrolled in plans with higher coinsurance rates. The reason is that, as noted above, the maximum out-of-pocket payments were related to income, so that lower-income families were more likely to exhaust their deductible or reach their out-of-pocket limit and thereafter get fully free care. This observation will turn out to be critical for the policy recommendations put forth later in this chapter.

A number of studies conducted since the RAND experiment have corroborated its finding that higher prices reduce health care use. Matthew Eichner, in a well-designed natural experiment using data from a fee-for-service plan from 1990 to 1992, found that the elasticity of health care spending ranged from 0.3 to 0.4—higher than, but still reasonably close to, the RAND estimate (Eichner 1997, 1998). Studies of the responsiveness of drug use to price have yielded similar results (Chandra, Gruber, and McKnight 2007).

It is possible that managed care, especially HMOs, could achieve many of the cost savings that would otherwise be achieved by cost sharing, thus blunting the impact. On the other hand, adding cost sharing to managed care could result in even more cost savings and possibly even a more sustainable complement of demand- and supply-side policies. These important questions have not been studied in any detail, but evidence from Eichner (1997) and other studies suggests that this may not be a major limitation, given that the responsiveness of health care spending to prices seems to have been similar in the early 1990s to what it was during the RAND experiment. Moreover, with strict managed care well below the levels it reached in the 1990s, this issue is less relevant today.

As already noted, the most significant limitation of the RAND experiment and subsequent studies is that they examined how individuals respond to greater cost sharing but by design did not examine the systemwide effects. Other research indicates that these effects could far exceed the direct effects on individual participants. A recent paper by Amy Finkelstein (2007) used the natural experiment provided by the introduction of Medicare in 1966 to infer the effect of expanding insurance—and thus reducing cost sharing—on health care spending. She compared the impact of Medicare in states such as Alabama, Kentucky, Mississippi, and Tennessee, whose residents had relatively limited insurance coverage before Medicare (the "treatment group"), with states such as Michigan and Ohio, whose residents had relatively extensive insurance coverage before Medicare (the "control group"). Finkelstein found that the systemwide effects of increased insurance on spending were six times larger than the individual effects in the RAND estimates. She further estimated that fully half of the increase in health expenditure from 1950 to 1990 resulted from the spread of health insurance and the consequent reduction in the out-of-pocket cost of health care.

Finkelstein (2007) explains why her systemwide natural experiment produced different results than RAND's more limited randomized trial: "I find that the introduction of Medicare is associated with substantial new hospital entry. I also find some suggestive evidence that Medicare's introduction is associated with increased adoption of cardiac technologies and increased spending on non-Medicare patients" (p. 3).

What might account for these associations? Finkelstein argues that the introduction of Medicare might have crossed an important demand threshold, making it a viable option for hospitals to undertake the fixed costs of entering new markets or buying expensive new equipment. In addition, the expansion of insurance might have altered broader cultural norms and specific practice with regard to which treatments are appropriate under which circumstances.

Over longer periods, cost sharing or its absence likely affects the incentive to develop technology (Weisbrod 1991). Relatively low cost sharing reduces demand for technologies that save money yet guarantees virtually unlimited demand for expensive new technologies. To use an improbable analogy, if automobile insurance covered the cost of gasoline, automakers would probably devote less research toward making cars more fuel efficient and devote more research toward improving acceleration, comfort, and other aspects of performance unrelated to gas prices. But an observer who sees only the current level of fuel-saving technology might fail to appreciate how much more fuel efficient cars could be if consumers had to pay out of pocket at the pump. As a result, cost sharing—through its impact on the invention and adoption of technology—has the potential to increase not only the level of spending, but also its growth rate. Over long periods, this effect grows more important.

More speculatively, some have claimed that greater cost sharing would improve the functioning of health care markets by stimulating both the availability of information about prices and consumer awareness of that information, putting consumers in a position to bargain for better prices.[18] There is little evidence for this proposition, although it is hard to test in the absence of the systemwide change that would create institutional mechanisms to present price and quality information that do not exist today. Moreover, there is reason to be skeptical that markets would function significantly better: insurance companies are very effective at bargaining for lower prices. For example, the largest type of health plan is the preferred provider organization, which bargains with providers over a fee schedule and uses the threat of expelling the provider from the network to enforce the lower prices. It is far from clear that consumers could do a better job bargaining. In fact, greater cost sharing could reduce the incentives that insurance companies have to bargain for lower prices because consumers would be picking up more of the higher prices.

Effects on Health Outcomes

Increased cost sharing has the potential to reduce health care spending substantially, whether it is going from free care to some cost sharing, or from

18. See, for example, John C. Goodman, "What Is Consumer-Directed Health Care? Comparing Patient Power with Other Decision Mechanisms," *Health Affairs*, web exclusive, October 24, 2006 (content.healthaffairs.org/cgi/reprint/25/6/w540).

some cost sharing to more cost sharing. But do these reductions come at the expense of good health outcomes?

According to the RAND team, the answer for a large majority of adults is clearly no: "Our results show that the 40 percent increase in services on the free-care plan had little or no measurable effect on health status for the average adult" (Newhouse and the Insurance Experiment Group 1993, p. 243). This conclusion applied to all middle- and high-income people and to low-income people in initially normal or good health. However, for an important minority of the population—the 6 percent of people who had both low incomes and initially poor health—shifting from free care to cost sharing did come at the expense of health outcomes.[19]

In interpreting the relevance of these results to public policy, it is important to emphasize that the RAND health plans linked maximum out-of-pocket payments to incomes, capping them at 5, 10, or 15 percent of income—or a fixed maximum amount. Thus low- and middle-income families were subject to less cost sharing than were high-income families. The RAND results do not support the claim that a fixed deductible, such as in an HSA-qualified plan, would leave health outcomes unchanged.

Health outcomes can be measured along several dimensions, including mortality (the probability of dying within some stated period) and quality of life (often proxied by the absence of disability or health-related restrictions on one's activity). Among all participants in the RAND study, mortality—or the predicted risk of dying—was virtually indistinguishable between free-care and cost-sharing plans. Disability actually improved with more cost sharing: the average number of restricted-activity days per year due to "illness, injury, medical treatment, or some other health problem" fell from an average of ten in the plan with free care to eight in the plan with the greatest cost sharing. Days lost from work also declined under the cost-sharing plans.

One of the strengths of the RAND experiment was the extraordinary level of medical detail tracked by the researchers. Their data included dozens of objective and subjective measures of health status in five general areas: "general health, including physical, mental, and social health; physiologic health (presence and effect of various chronic diseases); health habits; prevalence of symptoms and disability days; and risk of dying from

---

19. Even for this group, however, RAND found no evidence that going from some cost sharing to more cost sharing would reduce health outcomes. The samples used for this later comparison were, however, much smaller, making the finding less definitive than the comparisons between free care and cost sharing.

any cause related to various risk factors" (Newhouse and the Insurance Experiment Group 1993, p. 183). Here, however, the results were ambiguous: of thirty-two measures of health status, fifteen were better for people in the plan with free care, and seventeen were better in the plans with cost sharing. In most cases, however, the results were relatively close and were not statistically significantly better in either case.

For the sample as a whole, a summary general health index was slightly—but again not statistically significantly—better for people in the cost-sharing plans than for those in free care. The same was true for the subgroups of low-income people who were initially in good health and of high-income people regardless of their health status. The subjective results also favored the cost-sharing plans: participants were less likely to report health-related worries (for nine out of eleven conditions surveyed) or pain (for eight out of eleven) than participants in the free-care plan, although the differences were statistically insignificant.

These results on outcomes put the RAND finding on the equal reductions in "necessary" and "unnecessary" care in perspective. They suggest one of two possibilities: the "necessary" care itself was not very beneficial to health, or under free care, people consume more necessary, unnecessary, and flat-out harmful care. The net result is that health outcomes are not any better with more overall care than with less.

The RAND evidence finds that the relatively smaller effects associated with their randomized experiment do not harm health for most people. But if cost sharing were increased for everyone, then there would be systemwide effects that would likely lead to larger reductions in health spending. We do not have definitive evidence of the effects of these on health outcomes, but evidence from the introduction of Medicare is consistent with the general RAND result. Finkelstein and Robin McKnight (2005) found, on a wide range of indicators, no discernible impact of Medicare on elderly mortality from 1965 to 1975, despite its contribution to a 28 percent increase in medical spending. There are several reasons why this might be the case. First, before the introduction of Medicare, even the uninsured elderly had access to hospital treatment for the most serious treatable conditions. Those who could not pay usually received free care. Second, medical technology in the 1960s was inferior to that available today, thus Medicare did not immediately expand access to the full range of expensive but lifesaving treatments that are available today because many of those treatments did not yet exist. Third, the study only covered ten years, and some of the larger effects on mortality may have taken longer to materialize. Finally, the study assessed only mortality and not morbidity (the incidence of ill health among those who survive) or other health factors. In short, although the Medicare evidence is not completely applicable to health care in the twenty-first century, it does provide another indication that greater cost sharing need not worsen health.

The important exception to the generally favorable results in the RAND study was the subgroup consisting of low-income people in initially poor health (see Ku 2003; Hudman and O'Malley 2003). The 6 percent of people in this category fared worse with cost sharing in some significant ways. One was that people in this group were less likely to receive a diagnosis of hypertension and less likely to have the condition treated when they were subject to cost sharing. Because of this difference alone, members of this group who were in cost-sharing plans had a 10 percent higher rate of expected mortality. The same group of people was also somewhat less likely to have vision problems corrected and to have their dental cavities filled. Most other health indicators for this group were not affected by the level of cost sharing. Other studies have corroborated the negative effect of cost sharing on low-income populations. One study on the introduction of cost sharing among welfare recipients in Quebec found that cost sharing reduced therapeutic drug use, at the expense of a large increase in emergency room admissions and serious adverse events (Tamblyn and others 2001). Other studies, although less definitive, have also found that increasing cost sharing can result in the underuse of drugs by the chronically ill (Gibson, Ozminkowski, and Goetzel 2005; Goldman and others 2004; Thorpe 2006).

Because of the revolutionary changes in health care, the RAND results on health outcomes are considerably more difficult to generalize with confidence to the current health system than are the results on the responsiveness of health care spending to prices. In the late 1970s and early 1980s, there was considerably less that could be done to control hypertension. With today's drugs, the downside of not diagnosing hypertension could be far more consequential. Conversely, the advent and extensive use of expensive medical imaging technologies—such as computed tomography scans, ultrasound, magnetic resonance imaging, and nuclear medicine—might be a good example of "flat of the curve medicine" that has relatively little benefit at the margin and was not present in the RAND experiment.

Effects on Families' Financial Well-Being

The core function of any insurance is to protect against financial risk. Obviously, one direct effect of greater cost sharing in health insurance is to

Ftn. 20

impose greater financial risk on those insured.[20] The key question is whether the burden of this greater risk outweighs the potential savings for families through lower health care spending for a given level of health outcomes. The answer again turns out to depend on the income of the person subjected to cost sharing.

For example, critics of flawed cost-saving vehicles, such as the high-deductible health insurance plans associated with HSAs, correctly argue that they impose unaffordable out-of-pocket costs on those low-income families who fall ill. Supporters counter that "a number of features make HSA coverage potentially attractive to low-income workers. Premiums for high-deductible insurance are typically much lower than premiums for traditional coverage. That alone makes HSA-compatible coverage more affordable" (Cannon 2006, p.16). This would be a valid rebuttal were it not for the fact that a given increase in risk is less tolerable for a low-income family than it would be for a middle- or high-income family, and therefore the mere fact that high deductibles allow cheaper premiums avoids the real issue. The real issue is whether the savings from the lower premium are worth the added risk to families. In the case of low-income families, the answer to this question will often be no.

Consider a simple coin toss, where heads means winning $5,000 and tails means losing $5,000. The loss of $5,000 would be devastating for a family making only $10,000 a year, but much less of a problem for a family making $100,000. Suppose, further, that both families are allowed to demand compensation for submitting to the coin toss. The low-income family would probably require more compensation than the high-income family to willingly accept the bet. To put it differently, but in the end equivalently, a low-income family should be willing to pay more for insurance to protect against the risk of losing $5,000.

Now consider two hypothetical insurance plans offered to a nonelderly family: an insurance plan that covers all costs with no out-of-pocket payments (what economists call "complete insurance") and a typical high-deductible plan with a $4,000 deductible, 20 percent coinsurance, and a $6,000 out-of-pocket maximum. For simplicity of exposition, assume that both plans are actuarially fair, in the sense that the sum of premiums paid exactly equals in present value the expected total payout of health benefits,

---

20. The indirect effect depends on whether greater cost sharing for small costs leads more people to get insurance or to have insurance that limits large out-of-pocket risks. In this case, more cost sharing for smaller costs could end up reducing risks overall.

Table 7-6. Ex Post Outcomes for an Insured Family under Two Health Insurance Plans

Dollars

| | | High-deductible insurance[a] | |
Outcomes	Complete insurance (no out-of-pocket expenses)	Assuming fixed expenditures	Assuming a 5 percent across-the-board reduction in expenditures
Covered expenses	7,644	4,474	4,158
Average out-of-pocket	0	3,171	3,104
Average total cost	7,644	7,644	7,262
Minimum cost	7,644	4,474	4,158
Maximum cost	7,644	10,474	10,158
Percent of all participants with cost less than $7,644	...	47	51

Source: Author's calculations based on 2004 MEPS data.
a. Deductible = $4,000; coinsurance = 20 percent; maximum out-of-pocket expenses = $6,000.

and that there are no administrative costs or profits.[21] Table 7-6 compares total health care spending for an insured family under both plans. Spending under the high-deductible plan is calculated under two scenarios: the first assumes that health care expenditure in the aggregate is unchanged by the introduction of the cost-sharing plan, and the second assumes that the increased cost sharing lowers aggregate expenditure by 5 percent.[22]

In the first scenario, the premium for the high-deductible plan is more than $3,000 lower than that for the plan with full first-dollar coverage. Families with no medical expenses (the row labeled "minimum cost") would save the full difference. But families with very high medical expenses ("maximum cost") would end up about $3,000 worse off than under the complete insurance plan. The last row of the table uses data from the 2004 MEPS to estimate that, in total, about half of all plan participants would end up paying less under the high-deductible plan. If participants are risk averse, they would prefer the complete insurance plan.

21. These hypothetical premiums and the estimates derived from them are based on the distribution of health care spending in 2004, updated to 2006 levels using the growth of per capita health expenditures.

22. Equivalently, it could be assumed, for example, that health care expenditure falls by 20 percent and that, at the margin, $1 of health care expenditure is worth $0.75 in other spending. This would be roughly the case under the hypothesis that people are rational and consume extra health insurance because it is not counted in their taxable income.

Moreover, under relatively standard assumptions about risk aversion, the "cost" of the risk associated with the high-deductible plan (or, equivalently, the dollar amount needed to compensate for that risk) falls as income rises. Precise estimates of this cost depend on assumptions about people's attitude toward risk. Under one illustrative set of assumptions, a person with an annual income of $15,000 would require $1,300 in compensation for the added risk associated with the high-deductible plan, whereas a person with an annual income of $100,000 would require only $113 in compensation, and someone making $1 million would need a mere $11.[23]

Although the costs of the risk associated with greater cost sharing fall with income, the potential benefits are—to a first approximation—unrelated to income (where both quantities are measured in dollars). The principal benefit comes from a reduction in health care spending that is of little or no value; this is reflected in even lower premiums. To continue with our hypothetical example, assume that the introduction of the high-deductible plan reduces health care expenditure by 5 percent, and that the eliminated expenditure would have produced no additional health benefit and thus was of no value to the recipient. In this case, a fall in total health expenditures would further reduce the premium for the high-deductible plan, effectively saving the average participant an additional $400. In this simple example, this savings would be enough to more than compensate anyone making $35,000 or more for the risk associated with the high-deductible plan. Anyone making less than this amount would be worse off. Put another way, the high-deductible plan is like offering a coin toss with an asymmetrical payout: heads you win $3,500, tails you lose $2,500. Given risk aversion, this remains an undesirable gamble for many moderate-income families, but the higher one's income, the more likely one is to view this coin toss as a good bet.

Figure 7-6 extends this result by plotting both the cost of the added risk of the high-deductible plan (the curved line) and the benefit derived from lower health expenditure under that plan (the horizontal line) against income. It shows that shifting to the high-deductible plan imposes large losses on low-income households and provides somewhat smaller gains for high-income households.

---

23. These estimates assume a constant relative risk aversion, with a coefficient of relative risk aversion of 5. This is somewhat higher than the standard parameter value and is intended to be more consistent with people's revealed preferences about health insurance, which seem consistent with a higher degree of risk aversion, or with a completely different model such as loss aversion or mental accounts. See Rabin and Thaler (2001) for discussion.

Figure 7-6. Illustrative Costs and Benefits of a High-Deductible Plan

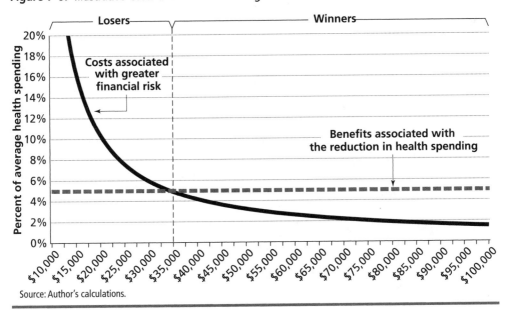

Source: Author's calculations.

Figure 7-6 is meant to illustrate a general principle, not to precisely calibrate the income cutoff at which higher cost sharing becomes beneficial. Any actual estimate would require much more accurate measures of the cost associated with a given level of risk, the amount by which the specified cost sharing would actually reduce health care spending, and the consequences of that reduced spending. If, contrary to RAND and other evidence, cost sharing achieves no reduction in spending, or reduces spending but thereby produces harmful health outcomes, the benefit line might fall to zero or even into negative territory. Then cost sharing would be a lose-lose proposition at all income levels: it would mean more risk and worse health outcomes for everyone.[24]

The scenario depicted in the figure is plausible, however, and the relationships are likely to be broadly similar across a range of assumptions about benefits and costs. In fact, the RAND evidence discussed above implies that the picture could look even worse for lower-income households

24. Strictly speaking, the correct test is not whether there is any deterioration in health outcomes but whether this deterioration is sufficiently worse that the extra money available for spending on other valued goods and services would not be enough to leave people better off.

because reducing their health care spending may worsen their health outcomes more than it does those of higher-income households. In that case, the horizontal line would become upward sloping, possibly even starting at or below zero on the left-hand side. That would strengthen the conclusions of this analysis. Conversely, it is conceivable that reductions in health care spending would be more valuable for lower-income households because the money saved would be more valuable to them in meeting their other needs. Put another way, given that health care spending, in total from all sources, now averages 80 percent of income for families below 125 percent of the poverty line and 8 percent of income for high-income families above 400 percent of poverty, it is conceivable that at the margin, shifting $1 out of health into other consumption would raise the low-income household's well-being more than it would raise that of the high-income household.

Effects of Income-Based Cost Sharing on Health Care Spending and Consumer Well-Being

The analysis thus far suggests that, ideally, cost sharing should be a function of income, and it should not be the same for all households. The evidence on the effects of cost sharing on health care spending (which are larger when cost sharing is related to income), on health outcomes (which were worse for chronically ill low-income people subjected to increased cost sharing), and on risk (a given degree of which is more costly for lower-income families) all points in this direction. This section explores further this concept of income-related cost sharing by simulating its effects on health care spending and overall economic welfare in the United States, using health care expenditure data from 2004.[25]

Simulation Method

The basic approach of the simulation method is to identify a set of insurance policies that differ in the degree and type of cost sharing and then calculate what each, if implemented for all the nonelderly with private insurance, would do to the price of health care and how much this change in price would affect the consumption of health care.[26] No attempt is made to

25. This analysis is similar to Feldstein and Gruber (1995), who used health care expenditure data from 1987. Note that 2004 data are adjusted to 2006 levels using the per capita growth in the corresponding aggregate.

26. In the income-related cost sharing plans, the percentage reductions in health spending would be somewhat smaller if the simulation included Medicaid beneficiaries because, unlike the privately insured population, they would see little if any reduction in their health expenditures.

treat different types of health care spending differently, to model what people's actual insurance plans are today, or to take into account the realistic case where people's health spending is spread out unpredictably throughout the year.

It turns out that the estimates depend crucially on how responsive health care spending is to changes in prices. Two possibilities are considered. The first uses the estimated elasticity from the RAND experiment, which found that a 10 percent increase in cost would lead to a 2.2 percent reduction in spending on health care. This can be interpreted as a short-run estimate that reflects immediate behavioral changes but ignores any longer-term, economywide responses such as the development and adoption of new medical technologies and practice styles. Alternatively, the RAND figure can be interpreted as an estimate of what would happen if only a minority of people were switched into a cost-sharing plan, so that the systemwide effects do not occur. (For example, in 2006 fewer than 5 percent of Americans had HSAs, and thus no systemwide effects are likely.)

As Finkelstein and other researchers have stressed, however, when change is systemwide, the effects can be substantially larger, even over a relatively brief five- to ten-year period. To account for this second possibility, the simulation also includes an alternative set of estimates intended to show what would happen if a 10 percent increase in the cost of health care led to a 6 percent reduction in spending. This is roughly half the elasticity found in the Finkelstein study.

The experiment thus analyzes several discrete scenarios, each of which assumes that a single insurance plan with a specific form of cost sharing is implemented nationwide.[27] The plans are as follows:

—A conventional plan with lower cost sharing. This plan is assumed to have a deductible of $350 for individuals ($700 for families) and 10 percent coinsurance up to an out-of-pocket maximum of $1,750 for individuals (or $3,500 for families).

—A high-deductible HSA plan. This plan is assumed to have a $2,000 deductible for individuals ($4,000 for families), 20 percent coinsurance, and a $3,000 ($6,000 for families) out-of-pocket maximum.

—A coinsurance rate of 50 percent up to 7.5 percent of income. Under this plan, households would pay half of their health care expenses up to

27. Of course, any real-world reform would allow for a much wider variety of plans. Unfortunately, the microdata do not provide any detail about cost sharing for each individual. As a result, this simulation follows the standard assumption of initially assigning everyone to the same plan. See, for example, Keeler and others (1996); Remler and Glied (2006); Feldstein and Gruber (1995).

7.5 percent of their income. From that point forward, insurance would pay 100 percent.

—A progressive cost-sharing plan. Under this plan, households would pay 50 percent coinsurance up to 7.5 percent of their income, except that families with incomes under 150 percent of the poverty line (about $30,000 for a family of four) would pay no coinsurance, and families with incomes between 150 and 200 percent of the poverty line would pay full coinsurance only up to 5 percent of their income and then would pay 7.5 percent coinsurance up to a maximum out-of-pocket cap at $15,000 (for a family earning $200,000).

As discussed earlier, under most existing insurance policies, cost sharing does not vary with income, and therefore cost sharing falls as a percentage of income as income rises. Under a universal health insurance system with income-sensitive cost sharing (such as the last two plans listed directly above), that would no longer be the case. In addition, no family would pay a substantial fraction of its income for out-of-pocket health care spending, unlike the current situation where many are uninsured, and many who are insured face unlimited liability for out-of-pocket expenses. All of the above plans cap out-of-pocket spending at some level. These plans are intended only as illustrative options for use in analyzing the broad issues raised by cost sharing. How to move in the direction suggested by the results of this simulation is discussed in a subsequent section.

Impact on Health Care Spending

Table 7-7 reports estimates of out-of-pocket health care spending, actuarially fair premiums, and total health care spending under each of the scenarios listed above. Several conclusions can be drawn.

Cost sharing can have a significant impact on total health care spending. Total health care spending falls by 13 to 32 percent in the scenarios. Even though the bulk of health care is purchased by a relatively small number of people with very high spending, enough spending takes place in the range affected by cost sharing to have a substantial effect. Under the HSA plan or the 7.5 percent income limit, about 80 percent of families would end the year with out-of-pocket expenses below the maximum, and thus would still be facing cost sharing at the margin. Whether this is good or bad, however, depends on the marginal benefits of this health spending.

Income-sensitive cost sharing can be more effective than one-size-fits-all cost sharing in reducing health care expenditures while minimizing the

Table 7-7. Simulated Health Care Spending under Alternative Policies and Moderate versus Strong Price Elasticity[a]

Units as indicated

Model	Spending (dollars)			Reduction (percent)	
	Out-of-pocket	Covered expenses (actuarially fair premium)	Total	In total premiums	In total spending
Assuming health-care spending responds moderately to price (elasticity = 0.22)					
Conventional plan	1,155	6,685	7,840		
HSA-type high-deductible plan	2,707	4,063	6,770	−34	−14
50 percent coinsurance up to 7.5 percent of income	1,916	4,833	6,748	−24	−14
Progressive cost-sharing plan	1,842	4,986	6,828	−22	−13
Assuming health-care spending responds strongly to price (elasticity = 0.6)					
Conventional plan	1,155	6,685	7,840		
HSA-type high-deductible plan	1,978	3,317	5,295	−44	−32
50 percent coinsurance up to 7.5 percent of income	1,398	3,899	5,296	−36	−32
Progressive cost-sharing plan	1,403	4,094	5,498	−34	−30

Source: Author's calculations.

a. Values may not sum to total because of rounding. Total premiums assume a load factor equal to 15 percent of the covered expenses in the conventional plan.

added financial risks. For example, both the HSA plan and the progressive cost-sharing plan result in similar reductions in spending: 14 percent and 13 percent, respectively, assuming a moderate responsiveness of spending to changes in price. Under the HSA plan, however, the average out-of-pocket payment is $2,707, compared with $1,842 under the plan with variable cost sharing.

The progressive cost-sharing plan would fully protect families under 150 percent of the poverty level from any out-of-pocket expenses, giving them better risk protection than most plans today. And it would have somewhat less cost sharing for families between 150 and 200 percent of poverty (and for families making above $200,000 to ensure that out-of-pocket maximums do not increase without limit). These protections come at virtually no aggregate cost—the percentage reduction in total health spending in the progressive cost-sharing plan is only 1 to 2 percentage points smaller than in the income-related cost-sharing plan. The reason is that the income-related cost-sharing plan has relatively little cost sharing for low-income families; reducing it still further has little overall effect on the plan.

Premiums fall by even more than total health expenditures, reducing an entry barrier to purchasing health insurance. All of the alternative plans would have two effects on premiums. First, they would reduce total health spending and thus required premiums. Second, they would increase out-of-pocket spending and thus, as a matter of accounting, would reduce the premiums needed to cover the remaining expenses. In the case of the progressive cost-sharing plan, for example, total health care spending would fall by 13 to 30 percent while total premiums would fall by 22 to 34 percent (after accounting for a loading charge that reflects administrative costs and profits).

It is better if the majority participates in the new plan than if only a minority participates. The reductions in health care spending are more than twice as large in the high price-responsiveness case, which corresponds to systemwide reform, than in the low price-responsiveness case.

Impact on Consumer Well-being

The ultimate goal of increased cost sharing is not simply to reduce health care spending or average out-of-pocket costs but to make people better off. Determining whether a given cost-sharing design makes people better off requires evaluating the trade-off between reduced spending and greater risk. That, in turn, depends on how people value both health care spending and financial risk. Both of these are much harder to quantify than the responsiveness of health care spending to prices, and therefore the estimates presented here are far less certain. Nevertheless, they strongly suggest that progressive cost sharing has the potential to provide robust protection against major risks and contribute to good health outcomes in a cost-effective manner.

Table 7-8 quantifies the risk associated with the alternative plans for families of four at different income levels, assuming that health spending responds moderately to prices (results are similar under the assumption that health spending responds more strongly to prices). The top half shows the standard deviation of out-of-pocket spending under the alternative plans. HSA-type plans increase the standard deviation of out-of-pocket spending for all incomes. In contrast, the progressive cost-sharing plan eliminates the volatility of out-of-pocket spending for near-poor families (making $25,000), reduces it for the moderate-income families (making $40,000), and increases it for middle- and high-income families. The bottom half shows a measure of the cost of risk associated with the four plans, expressed as a percentage of average health spending in the

Table 7-8. Financial Risks of Alternative Plans for a Family of Four

Units as indicated

Plan type	Risk at family income of			
	$25,000	$40,000	$80,000	$250,000
Standard deviation of out-of-pocket spending (dollars)				
Conventional plan	783	783	783	783
HSA-type high-deductible plan	1,915	1,915	1,915	1,915
50 percent coinsurance up to 7.5 percent of income	637	1,077	2,055	4,087
Progressive cost-sharing plan	0	681	2,052	3,697
Cost of risk (as a percent of health spending)				
Conventional plan	0.7	0.4	0.2	0.1
HSA-type high-deductible plan	3.6	2.2	1.1	0.4
50 percent coinsurance up to 7.5 percent of income	0.4	0.7	1.3	1.8
Progressive cost-sharing plan	0.0	0.3	1.3	1.4

Source: Author's calculations assuming moderate responsiveness of health spending to prices.

base case.[28] With the HSA-type plan, the cost of risk is substantially higher for low-income families because they are the most averse to the potential losses. Under the progressive cost-sharing plan, low- and moderate-income families face a lower cost of risk than under conventional insurance plans. Middle-income families face a level of risk similar to what they face under HSAs, and high-income families face more risk.

All three alternatives create somewhat more risk for middle- and upper-income families. But they also save these families substantial sums on premiums. On average, they would save these families an equivalent of 13 to 14 percent of their total health spending, allowing families to spend more on other valued goods and services such as housing, food, clothing, and even entertainment. Are these savings enough to justify the risks? For low- and moderate-income families under the progressive cost-sharing plan the answer is obviously yes: these families save money *and* face less risk.[29]

28. Like the earlier discussion, this assumes a coefficient of relative risk aversion of 5. This is higher than standard estimates of risk aversion, but as noted earlier, it may correspond more accurately to the way people appear to behave in response to the risk of increased out-of-pocket health care expenses.

29. Note that the implicit assumption in table 7-8 is that all families pay a premium that reflects their maximum out-of-pocket expenses. In other words, it assumes that lower-income families pay a higher premium because they have a lower out-of-pocket limit. If premiums were equal for all families, then in addition to the other effects, there would also be a substantial redistribution from higher-income families to lower-income families.

Under the HSA-plan the answer is much more equivocal: these families face more risks, and the evidence from RAND and subsequent studies suggests that these families could also face significant health risks. For middle- and high-income families, the evidence from the RAND study strongly suggests that the savings of 13 to 14 percent of total health spending will come at virtually no cost in terms of health, more than repaying the added financial risks.

For Some, Income-Related Cost Sharing Could Reduce Financial Risk and Increase Health Care Spending

This analysis assumes that the entire population is shifted from a conventional insurance plan with a $1,750 ($3,500 for families) out-of-pocket maximum to a plan that may have more cost sharing, depending on the person's income. In reality, many people today are uninsured or underinsured. Income-related cost sharing will unambiguously reduce the price of their health care, reduce the financial risk they face, and increase their health care spending. In total, 22 percent of workers have insurance plans that expose them to unlimited liability.[30] In contrast, the progressive cost-sharing plan would have out-of-pocket limits for all families, providing more financial protection against major risks and probably contributing to better health outcomes. Even HSA-qualified insurance plans are required to have an out-of-pocket limit no greater than $5,500 for an individual and $11,000 for a family, making them better at minimizing major health risks than some of the insurance plans on the market today.

Other Important Considerations in Designing Effective Cost Sharing

Further refinements in the design of cost sharing can have additional positive effects on the health care system. One such refinement would be to exempt from cost sharing certain types of health care that have been well documented to be particularly beneficial. This kind of "smart," evidence-based cost sharing can improve the delivery of health care, particularly of health care for the chronically ill.

Evidence-Based Cost Sharing

As the RAND study, the evidence from the large disparities in Medicare spending across counties, and other findings demonstrate, we can achieve

---

30. Some of these workers are in HMOs with little cost sharing, though, so this exposure does not represent a general risk.

health outcomes equally good as we are getting today for substantially less money and with substantially fewer treatments. In many cases, American health care is being practiced on what is called the "flat of the curve," with little marginal health benefit for additional spending and treatments. There are many important exceptions, however. In those cases, indiscriminate, across-the-board cost sharing is likely to make people worse off. The RAND experiment identified some important exceptions involving low-income people with chronic conditions. According to Joseph Newhouse and the Insurance Experiment Group (1993, p. 351), all of these conditions shared three characteristics:

—"The conditions in question are relatively common.

—"The standard diagnostic tests for these conditions are relatively inexpensive (for example, measuring blood pressure, giving a vision refraction test, taking an x-ray of a tooth).

—"The standard treatment is well known, inexpensive, and more effective than the standard treatments for many other medical conditions."

Newhouse goes on to note that it would be easy to carve dental care and vision care out of the broader health care system and institute cost sharing for them separately. Hypertension is harder to carve out because it is normally diagnosed and treated by the same medical professionals who provide most other health care, and as part of the same process. Even with hypertension, though, the RAND experiment found that blood pressure screening alone provided half the total benefit of free care at a fraction of the total cost. Moreover, once individuals knew that they were hypertensive, there was little difference in treatment between those receiving free care and those with cost sharing.

The rules under which high-deductible plans qualify as HSAs are designed with some of these lessons in mind. HSAs are allowed to provide first-dollar coverage for preventive services, thus exempting these from cost sharing. Prevention is defined to include "periodic health evaluations . . . such as annual physicals, routine pre-natal and well-child care, child and adult immunizations, tobacco cessation programs, obesity weight-loss programs, screening services" (Department of the Treasury 2004). In 2006, 82 percent of workers enrolled in HSA-qualified high-deductible plans had at least some cost-sharing exemptions for preventive services (Kaiser 2006). The current exceptions under HSAs may be inadequate, however, because they relate only to preventive care, including screenings. They fail to address disease management for the high-risk insured and the chronically ill, including diabetics, people with high cholesterol, people with a history of heart disease, and depression.

There is substantial evidence that high-risk individuals and the chronically ill underutilize care, and there is some evidence that cost sharing could make the problem worse. With respect to these issues, policymakers and the insurance industry are focusing most of their attention on the supply side: providers are encouraged to apply more evidence-based care, through techniques ranging from better dissemination of information to pay-for-performance rules, which reimburse providers on the basis of health care inputs used or even outcomes. These supply-side measures could, however, be complemented by demand-side measures that relate cost sharing to medical evidence (Fenwick, Claxton, and Sculpher 2001). In a sense, utilization review already does this by requiring people to pay in full for denied health treatments (that is, 100 percent coinsurance). But for plans where cost sharing is the norm, the goal would be to carve out exceptions based on the best evidence. Such exceptions would not just lower the relative price of certain services; they would also send a strong signal about the effectiveness of those services, thus complementing the supply-side measures.

The devil, of course, is in the details, and our current state of knowledge is very poor about both links in the chain: how cost sharing (including differential cost sharing) affects the use of different types of health care and how health care affects health outcomes. We simply do not know enough to design an effective system of exceptions. Additional research would help. The best evidence remains the RAND Health Insurance Experiment, but it was launched more than thirty years ago, when health technology and health insurance were very different from what they are today. Although subsequent studies have generally corroborated its results, the confidence that we should have in approaching such an important issue is still lacking. Further research into which health measures should be cost free for consumers is critical; another round of RAND-like experiments would repay its cost several hundredfold. Yet even if we had perfect knowledge about what conditions should be exempted from cost sharing, a substantial political risk would remain. Decisions might be influenced not by solid medical evidence alone but also by political pressure from medical providers.

There are two possible ways to deal with both of these problems. The first is to establish a respected national board, such as Britain's National Institute for Health and Clinical Excellence, to promulgate standards not just for treatment but also for evidence-based cost sharing and other aspects of the demand side of health insurance. The second way would be to give insurance companies some flexibility to experiment with their own designs for evidence-based cost sharing, possibly by allowing them broad exceptions but then putting a percentage limit on the services they may exempt. The resulting competition and freedom of choice might help in arriving at a better recipe. At the very least, it would give researchers and policymakers more information to use in designing more effective cost-sharing regimes.

Ultimately, any such change would offset some of the spending reductions from the greater cost sharing, but substantial savings are likely to remain. Lambrew, for example, estimates that total prevention spending is $70 billion, or 3 percent of total health spending.[31] Carving this spending out, either through Lambrew's proposed Wellness Trust or through smart cost sharing, would have only a small impact on the analysis discussed above. Carving out drugs to manage chronic conditions would be somewhat more important but still would not undo the benefits of lower premiums. For example, exempting all drugs from the progressive cost-sharing plan and instead treating them as they are under insurance today would lead to a reduction in total health spending of 10 percent instead of 13 percent.

Insurance for the Chronically Ill

The other major shortcoming of increased cost sharing is its effect on the chronically ill. In effect, the earlier discussion of risk assumed that medical risks are of a one-time nature: an individual policyholder might fall ill and receive insurance payouts one year but be in good health again the next and receive nothing. But insurance also covers—and should cover—the cost of chronic illness. Unlike those who suffer an acute illness and then return to full health, the insured who are chronically ill are quite likely to receive more in insurance payouts than they contribute over a period that can extend into many decades. Health insurance thus redistributes resources from the usually healthy to the chronically ill. In a just and equitable society, this is seen as a good thing, but increasing cost sharing undoes some of the extra support that the chronically ill receive. It puts a greater financial burden on many of the chronically ill than they can or should bear.

The issue is a serious one and requires a response. Smarter, evidence-based cost sharing could help by providing more first-dollar coverage for treatments known to be highly effective in managing chronic illness. In such cases, presumably, there is little overuse of care, and thus removing the price

31. See chapter 8 in this volume.

signal has little downside, while the insurance itself provides protection against financial risk on the upside (Chandra, Gruber, and McKnight 2007).

Other measures should also be considered, including income tax credits for people who reach their out-of-pocket limit year after year. Although potentially complicated to administer, such a measure would make the redistribution from the healthy to the chronically ill more transparent. It would also offer greater assurance that such redistribution will continue, compared with the risk-pooling mechanisms under the current system that are fragmenting and may collapse.

Finally, as argued above, greater cost sharing would ideally be implemented as part of a broader health reform that includes universal coverage. Any such reform should also include other measures—such as new pooling options, community rating, guaranteed renewal, reinsurance, and risk-adjusted vouchers—that could improve the availability and effectiveness of insurance for the chronically ill.

Anything that helps provide insurance for the chronically ill will also reduce the extent of adverse selection, the process by which healthier people opt into plans with higher cost sharing, leaving sicker people in plans with lower cost sharing. Adverse selection is a problem not just because of the need for equity but also because it can result in market failures that lead people into the wrong insurance plans or even cause some types of desirable insurance plans to cease to exist.

Implementing Better Cost Sharing

In practice, a number of impediments stand in the way of the health insurance market developing income-related cost sharing on its own. For one thing, it would be difficult for private insurance companies to develop and administer policies that have different cost sharing for families with different incomes, especially in the context of an employer-sponsored system. Furthermore, the current tax code is biased toward plans with lower cost sharing: it allows employees to exclude employer contributions to their health insurance premiums from their taxable income but does not allow a corresponding deduction of their out-of-pocket health care expenses.[32] This bias also reduces the transparency of health premiums, masking the trade-off between health care spending and spending on all other goods. All else equal, no one would choose a plan with higher cost sharing, and

---

32. Exceptions include flexible spending accounts and out-of-pocket expenses exceeding 7.5 percent of income, although this applies only for people that itemize their deductions.

all else equal, no one would choose a plan with a higher premium. However, if insured workers observe their own out-of-pocket expenses but do not observe the premiums they pay indirectly because the payment takes the form of lower wages, it is harder to make this trade-off.

Another reason people end up in insurance plans that do not provide coverage against major risks is that health care providers—primarily hospitals and physicians—often simply write off large, uncovered expenses that the patient cannot or will not pay. This weakens the demand for insurance to cover these major risks. Finally, there may be significant behavioral obstacles in the way people understand insurance, especially for small risks. The following subsection discusses some possible strategies to overcome these obstacles and move closer to a system of cost sharing that minimizes major financial risks and improves health outcomes in a cost-effective manner.

How to Make Cost Sharing Income-Sensitive

The simplest and cleanest way to implement income-related cost sharing would be as part of a far-reaching fundamental health reform. For instance, a single-payer insurance system could easily incorporate income-related cost sharing, either in the form of a 7.5-percent-of-income limit on out-of-pocket expenses or with different tiers of cost sharing for different income groups. Alternatively, a system of risk-adjusted vouchers, such as that proposed by Victor Fuchs and Ezekiel Emanuel (2005), could include income-related cost sharing in the benefit mandate for private insurance companies under the proposal.[33] As discussed earlier, the potential benefits of greater cost sharing will be larger if the change is systemwide.

Another option would be for the federal government to start by introducing income-sensitive cost sharing into its own programs, such as Medicare, or as part of the Federal Employee Health Benefits Program, which covers about 9 million current and former government workers and their dependents (Government Accountability Office 2006). The government could also encourage private insurance companies to offer income-related coinsurance, possibly by limiting the current tax exclusion to employers that purchase plans with this feature. Alternatively, the government could implement income-sensitive cost sharing directly, with a tax credit for out-of-pocket medical expenses in excess of a certain fraction of

---

33. See also Emanuel and Fuchs, chapter 4 in this volume, for their proposal of a voucher system.

income. This approach, however, raises serious issues of complexity and the timing of payments (Department of the Treasury 1977; Seidman 1980).[34]

Income-related coinsurance would entail some additional administrative complexities, but the potential gains are so large that it is worth the effort to try to overcome them. It is certainly feasible to do so; the RAND experiment implemented income-related cost sharing in the mid-1970s. Doing it at scale and with today's superior information technology would be easier. Moreover, income-related cost sharing already exists to a limited degree in Medicaid, the State Children's Health Insurance Program, and a handful of private plans. Any additional administrative costs would be well worth the expected benefits. The alternatives, in contrast, are not very desirable: limiting cost sharing for everyone is an inefficient way to protect the low-income, chronically ill minority, and imposing an aggressive form of cost sharing on everyone would harm the most vulnerable.

Income-Related Compensation

Income-related compensation could be an administratively simpler alternative to income-related coinsurance. Assume, for example, that every family in the country was enrolled in a plan with a $4,000 deductible. Families could then receive matching funds or tax credits from the government to offset their payments against this deductible, and the contributions could be inversely proportional to income. Or, equivalently, lower-income households could receive a larger subsidy on their premium payments than higher-income households, as Medicare is now starting to do.

But income-related compensation would not be as efficient or desirable as income-related coinsurance, for two reasons. First, it would not change the incentives to consume health care. Income-related premiums in Medicare, for example, are a form of progressive tax financing for the program, but they are effectively a sunk cost that does not affect further spending. Second, the RAND study and other evidence indicate that low-income individuals and the chronically ill may end up worse off if they are forced to pay substantial amounts out of pocket. Specifically, the RAND experiment found no evidence that the income effect associated with compensation would lead to higher health spending and thus remedy the problem.

Notably, HSAs have the opposite effect of income-related compensation. They provide larger tax breaks for higher-income families that can afford to save more and are in higher tax brackets; these families thus benefit

---

34. The credit would presumably be claimable only once a year, on the taxpayer's annual income tax return.

more from the tax-free accumulation of interest on those savings. So not only do HSAs impose more risk on the lower-income families who can least afford it, but they also get the compensation for this risk backward.

Reforming the Tax Treatment of Health Insurance

Another way to increase cost sharing and improve the cost-effectiveness of health insurance involves reforming the tax treatment of health insurance. The excludability of employer contributions to health insurance would be limited or eliminated and replaced with a progressive tax credit or voucher.[35] Eliminating the tax advantage of premiums over out-of-pocket payments in this way would encourage more cost sharing, which, moreover, would be economywide, magnifying the benefits due to the systemic effects of any reform. In addition, turning the regressive deduction into a progressive credit would effectively compensate low- and moderate-income households for the cost of the additional risk they would bear under increased cost sharing.

Done the wrong way, however, changing the tax treatment could be more damaging than beneficial. If this reform extended the tax benefits to the purchase of health insurance in the individual market, then it would be critical to also put in place complementary reforms to prevent the employer-sponsored system from unraveling without creating a sound pooling mechanism in its place. Plans that lack this safeguard risk—such as the Bush administration's proposal—would result in substantial numbers of people losing their health insurance as employers drop coverage.[36]

Encouraging Greater Transparency

Finally, greater transparency about the trade-off between health care spending and spending on other goods and services could make a helpful difference in reducing the former or improving the ways in which it is spent. Everyone wants lower premiums, no out-of-pocket outlays, and unlimited access to specialists, high-technology tests, and expensive treatments. Ultimately, however, the trade-offs between these conflicting desires must be acknowledged. It is to the advantage of us all to understand that we pay for health care in four ways: direct outlays, insurance premiums, lower wages, and higher taxes. In the absence of such awareness, increased cost sharing will be misperceived as shifting costs to individual consumers

---

35. Butler (1991) was an early proponent of this.

36. See Furman (2006a) and Burman and others (2007) for a more detailed discussion of how to transform the tax exclusion without disrupting pooling mechanisms.

while providing a windfall to insurers, health providers, or other groups, rather than potentially increasing one type of consumer payment while reducing another type of consumer payment by even more.

Conclusions

The extent to which individual consumers bear the cost of the health care they receive clearly influences overall health care spending. Over the past four decades, large relative reductions in cost sharing have contributed to a steady increase in total health care expenditure. Reversing some of that decline could help bring health costs down, freeing up resources to spend on more highly valued goods and services—perhaps including other, more beneficial kinds of health care—with little or no adverse impact on health outcomes. Undoing some of the reduction in cost sharing could also bring down the cost of health insurance, reducing the number of uninsured. Finally, exposure to smaller risks—but caps on bigger risks—could improve financial security, both directly by limiting large health bills and indirectly by making insurance more affordable and thus more sustainable.

Increased cost sharing for small risks while protecting against large risks is not, however, a panacea. Instead, it is one dimension of a difficult trade-off, the other being the financial risk of high out-of-pocket health care expenses. For some, including families below or near the poverty line and the bulk of Medicaid beneficiaries, the trade-off is probably not worth it. These families should be largely shielded from cost sharing. But, for the majority of households, adding small risks is worth the savings, especially if cost sharing—or the associated compensation—can be related to income and any changes are made in a "smart" way that improves health outcomes.

Like any major public policy—especially one designed to reduce health care spending—increased cost sharing will produce winners and losers. But far from derailing such reform, this should be an impetus to reformers to be careful about the way in which cost sharing is implemented and to make adjustments as the emerging evidence warrants. For example, we already know it is much cheaper to protect low-income individuals from the health consequences of hypertension by providing free blood pressure screenings than it is to offer free care for all. Smart cost sharing can be tailored to keep such beneficial interventions cost free—and therefore widely used—while achieving the goal of cost containment.

No health care system is perfect. Trying to provide complete, first-to-last-dollar protection for everyone would be expensive and unrealistic. Moreover, attempts at complete first-to-last-dollar protection have been accompanied by the imposition of stricter controls on use by insurance companies—and that has not proven popular with much of the public. Increased cost sharing at least has the merit of giving individuals greater control over tough choices.

Increased cost sharing can be part of a very good health care system. It would be a critical step forward, freeing up funds to fix the other chronic problems that plague the system, in particular the plight of the tens of millions who are uninsured or underinsured. It could be imaginatively designed to steer health care spending to where it is most effective. In short, progressive cost sharing could be an integral part of a reformed health care system that, while far from perfect, would be better than what we currently have—and moving in the right direction.

References

Aaron, Henry J., William B. Schwartz, and Melissa Cox. 2005. *Can We Say No: The Challenge of Rationing Health Care.* Brookings.

Agency for Healthcare Research and Quality. 1987. *National Medical Expenditure Survey.* Rockville, Md.: U.S. Department of Health and Human Services.

Artiga, Samantha, and Molly O'Malley. 2005. "Increasing Premiums and Cost Sharing in Medicaid and SCHIP: Recent State Experiences." Issue Paper 7322. Washington: Kaiser Commission on Medicaid and the Uninsured.

Bureau of Labor Statistics. Various years. *Consumer Expenditure Survey.*

Burman, Leonard, and others. 2007. "An Evaluation of the President's Health Insurance Proposal." *Tax Notes* 114, no. 10.

Butler, Stuart M. 1991. "A Tax Reform Strategy to Deal with the Uninsured." *Journal of the American Medical Association* 265, no. 19: 2541–44.

Cannon, Michael F. 2006. "Health Savings Accounts: Do the Critics Have a Point?" Policy Analysis 569. Washington: Cato Institute.

Chandra, Amitabh, Jonathan Gruber, and Robin McKnight. 2007. "Patient Cost Sharing, Hospitalization Offsets, and the Design of Optimal Health Insurance for the Elderly." Working Paper 12972. Cambridge, Mass.: National Bureau of Economic Research.

Cogan, John F., Glenn R. Hubbard, and Daniel P. Kessler. 2005. *Healthy, Wealthy, and Wise: Five Steps to a Better Health Care System.* Washington: American Enterprise Institute.

Collins, Sara R. 2006. "Health Savings Accounts: Why They Won't Cure What Ails U.S. Health Care." Testimony before Committee on Ways and Means, House of Representatives. New York: Commonwealth Fund (June 28).

Committee on the Consequences of Uninsurance. 2003. *Hidden Costs, Value Lost: Uninsurance in America.* Washington: Institute of Medicine.

Cutler, David M., Allison B. Rosen, and Sandeep Vijan. 2006. "The Value of Medical Spending in the United States, 1960–2000." *New England Journal of Medicine* 355 (9): 920–27.

DeNavas-Walt, Carmen, Bernadette D. Proctor, and Jessica Smith. 2007. *Income, Poverty, and Health Insurance Coverage in the United States: 2006.* U.S. Census Bureau, Current Population Reports, P60-233. (Government Printing Office, 2007).

Eichner, Matthew Jason. 1997. "Medical Expenditures and Major Risk Health Insurance." Doctoral dissertation, Massachusetts Institute of Technology.

————. 1998. "The Demand for Medical Care: What People Pay Does Matter." *American Economic Review* 88, no. 2: 117–21.

Feldstein, Martin S. 1971. "A New Approach to National Health Insurance." *Public Interest,* no. 23: 93–105.

Feldstein, Martin S., and Jonathan Gruber. 1995. "A Major Risk Approach to Health Insurance Reform." In *Tax Policy and the Economy,* vol. 9, edited by James Poterba, pp. 103–30. MIT Press.

Fenwick, Elisabeth, Karl Claxton, and Mark Sculpher. 2001. "Representing Uncertainty: The Role of Cost-Effectiveness Acceptability Curves." *Health Economics* 10, no. 8:779–87.

Finkelstein, Amy. 2007. "The Aggregate Effects of Health Insurance: Evidence from the Introduction of Medicare." *Quarterly Journal of Economics* 122, no. 1: 1–37.

Finkelstein, Amy, and Robin McKnight. 2005. "What Did Medicare Do (and Was It Worth It)?" Working Paper 1609. Cambridge, Mass.: National Bureau of Economic Research (September).

Fisher, Elliott S. 2003. "Medical Care: Is More Always Better?" *New England Journal of Medicine* 349, no. 17: 1665–67.

Fuchs, Victor R., and Ezekiel J. Emanuel. 2005. "Health Care Vouchers: A Proposal for Universal Coverage." *New England Journal of Medicine* 352, no. 12: 1255–60.

Furman, Jason. 2006a. "Our Unhealthy Tax Code." *Democracy Journal* no. 1 (Summer): 45–56.

————. 2006b. "Two Wrongs Do Not Make a Right." *National Tax Journal* 59, no. 3: 491–508.

Gibson, Teresa B., Ronald J. Ozminkowski, and Ron Z. Goetzel. 2005. "The Effects of Prescription Drug Cost Sharing: A Review of the Evidence." *American Journal of Managed Care* 11, no. 11: 730–40.

Goldman, Dana P., and others. 2004. "Pharmacy Benefits and the Use of Drugs by the Chronically Ill." *Journal of the American Medical Association* 291, no. 19: 2344–50.

Gruber, Jonathan. 1994. "The Incidence of Mandated Maternity Benefits." *American Economic Review* 84, no. 3: 622–41.

————. 2006. "The Role of Consumer Copayments for Health Care: Lessons from the RAND Health Insurance Experiment and Beyond." Report 7566. Menlo Park, Calif.: Kaiser Family Foundation.

Hall, Robert E., and Charles I. Jones. 2007. "The Value of Life and the Rise in Health Spending." *Quarterly Journal of Economics* 122, no. 1: 39–72.

Henderson, James W. 2005. *Health Economics and Policy with Economic Applications.* 3d ed. Mason, Ohio: South-Western College Publishing.

Hudman, Julie, and Molly O'Malley. 2003. *Health Insurance Premiums and Cost Sharing: Findings from the Research on Low-Income Populations.* Kaiser Commission on Medicaid and the Uninsured, Menlo Park, Calif. (April).

Kaiser Family Foundation, the Health Research and Educational Trust, and the Center for Studying Health System Change. 2006. *Employer Health Benefits: 2006 Annual Survey.* Washington.

Keeler, Emmett B., and others. 1996. "Can Medical Savings Accounts for the Nonelderly Reduce Health Care Costs?" *Journal of the American Medical Association* 275, no. 21: 1666–71.

Ku, Leighton. 2003. "Charging the Poor More for Health Care: Cost Sharing in Medicaid." Report. Washington: Center on Budget and Policy Priorities.

Ku, Leighton, and Victoria Wachino. 2005. "The Effect of Increased Cost Sharing in Medicaid: A Summary of Research Findings." Report. Washington: Center on Budget and Policy Priorities.

Manning, Willard G., and others. 1987. "Health Insurance and the Demand for Medical Care: Evidence from a Randomized Experiment." *American Economic Review* 77, no. 3: 251–77.

McGlynn, Elizabeth A. 1998. "Assessing the Appropriateness of Care: How Much Is Too Much?" Research Brief RB-4522. Santa Monica, Calif.: RAND.

Murphy, Kevin M., and Robert H. Topel. 2006. "The Value of Health and Longevity." *Journal of Political Economy* 114, no. 5: 871–904.

National Center for Health Services Research. 1977. *National Medical Care Expenditure Survey,* Hyattsville, Md.

Newhouse, Joseph P. 2004. "Consumer-Directed Health Plans and the RAND Health Insurance Experiment." *Health Affairs* 23, no. 6: 107–13.

Newhouse, Joseph P., and the Insurance Experiment Group. 1993. *Free for All? Lessons from the RAND Health Insurance Experiment.* Harvard University Press.

Organization for Economic Cooperation and Development (OECD). 2006. OECD *Health Data 2006: A Comparative Analysis of 30 Countries.* CD-ROM or Internet subscription database. Paris.

Rabin, Matthew, and Richard H. Thaler. 2001. "Anomalies: Risk Aversion." *Journal of Economic Perspectives* 15, no. 1: 219–32.

Remler, Dahlia K., and Sherry A. Glied. 2006. "How Much More Cost Sharing Will Health Savings Accounts Bring?" *Health Affairs* 25, no. 4: 1070–78.

Rice, Thomas, and Kenneth E. Thorpe. 1993. "Income-Related Cost Sharing in Health Insurance." *Health Affairs* 12, no. 1: 21–39.

Seidman, Laurence S. 1980. "Income-Related Cost Sharing: A Strategy for the Health Sector." In *National Health Insurance: What Now, What Later, What Never?* edited by Mark V. Pauly, pp. 307–28. Washington: AEI Press.

Tamblyn, Robyn, and others. 2001. "Adverse Events Associated with Prescription Drug Cost-Sharing among Poor and Elderly Persons." *Journal of the American Medical Association* 285, no. 4: 421–29.

Thorpe, Kenneth E. 2006. "Cost Sharing, Caps on Benefits, and the Chronically Ill: A Policy Mismatch." *New England Journal of Medicine* 354, no. 22: 2385–86.

U.S. Department of the Treasury. 1977. *Blueprints for Basic Tax Reform.* Government Printing Office.

———. 2004. "Provides a Safe Harbor for Preventive Care Benefits." Notice 2004-23.

U.S. Government Accountability Office. 2006. *Federal Employees Health Benefits Program First-Year Experience with High-Deductible Health Plans and Health Savings Accounts.* GAO-06-271.

Weisbrod, Burton A. 1991. "The Health Care Quadrilemma: An Essay on Technological Change, Insurance, Quality of Care, and Cost Containment." *Journal of Economic Literature* 29, no. 2: 523–52.

A Wellness Trust to Prioritize Disease Prevention

8

JEANNE M. LAMBREW

T he health challenges faced at the beginning of the twenty-first century are different from and, in some ways, more daunting than those at the turn of the twentieth century. There were considerable gains made over the last century; for example, life expectancy has lengthened by thirty years and infant mortality has dropped by 90 percent (Centers for Disease Control and Prevention [CDC] 1999). Public health and medicine combined to reduce infectious disease. No longer are diseases like tuberculosis, influenza, and pneumonia the major killers that they were in 1900 (see figure 8-1). In addition, rapid scientific advances have largely converted diseases like HIV/AIDS from acute and deadly illnesses into chronic ones in the United States.

Growing Preventable Disease Burden

Chronic diseases are this century's epidemic. Five chronic diseases—cardiovascular disease, stroke, cancer, chronic obstructive pulmonary disease, and diabetes—account for two-thirds of all deaths in the United States

The ideas in this paper were informed by colleagues at the Center for American Progress, especially John Podesta and Meredith King. Additional thanks are extended to the panel of reviewers who helped sharpen the ideas.

Figure 8-1. Shift toward Chronic Disease, 1900 and 2003

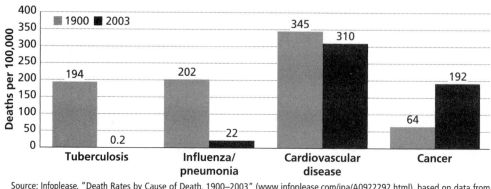

Source: Infoplease, "Death Rates by Cause of Death, 1900–2003" (www.infoplease.com/ipa/A0922292.html), based on data from the U.S. Public Health Service and the U.S. National Center for Health Statistics.

(CDC 2004b). An estimated 45 percent of Americans (125 million) had a chronic illness in 2000. This is projected to rise to 50 percent (157 million) by 2020 (Wu and Green 2000; see figure 8-2). The elderly are particularly prone to chronic illness: an estimated 87 percent of Medicare beneficiaries have at least one chronic illness (Kaiser Family Foundation 2005). One study found that virtually all of the spending growth in Medicare over the past fifteen years resulted from increased spending on people with multiple chronic conditions.[1]

While cardiovascular disease has been a long-standing cause of death, a particularly troubling trend has been the increase in diabetes. The number of people with diabetes has doubled in the past fifteen years, and one in three persons born in 2000 can expect to have diabetes in his or her lifetime (CDC 2006a). Certain racial and ethnic minorities are particularly vulnerable: the rate of diabetes is 50 to 80 percent higher among African Americans than it is among non-Hispanic whites.

Much of the morbidity—in some cases, mortality—associated with this growing chronic disease burden is preventable. The CDC estimates that tobacco use remains the main risk factor leading to deadly disease (Mokdad and others 2004; see figure 8-3). Compared to nonsmokers, smokers are

1. Kenneth E. Thorpe and David H. Howard, "The Rise in Spending among Medicare Beneficiaries: The Role of Chronic Disease Prevalence and Changes in Treatment Intensity," *Health Affairs,* web exclusive, August 22, 2006 (content.healthaffairs.org/cgi/content/abstract/25/5/w378).

Figure 8-2. Projected Prevalence of Chronic Disease, 2000 and 2020

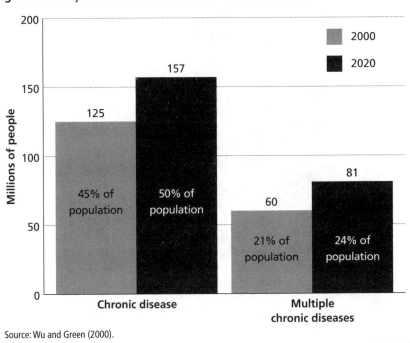

Source: Wu and Green (2000).

twelve to twenty-four times more likely to develop lung cancer, ten times more likely to die from chronic obstructive pulmonary disease, and two to four times more likely to develop coronary heart disease (CDC 2004a). However, poor diet and physical inactivity have risen as causes of death and could surpass tobacco use in the next decade. About 24 percent of Americans were obese in 2005, up from 15 percent in 1995 (CDC 2006c). Obesity contributes to a wide range of chronic conditions, from diabetes to stroke to cancer. One study estimates that as a result of obesity, a twenty-year-old man could experience a 17 percent reduction in life expectancy (Fontaine and others 2003). If trends continue, children's life spans may be shorter than those of their parents for the first time in about a century (Olshansky and others 2005).

Unlike some health care challenges, knowledge exists about ways to curtail chronic illness as well as some of the lingering infectious diseases. Disease prevention and health promotion are broadly defined as actions to prevent the onset of disease (primary prevention) and to detect and treat disease in its early stages (secondary prevention). Prevention delivered

Figure 8-3. Causes of Death in the United States, 2000

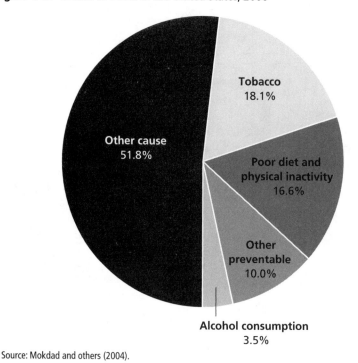

Source: Mokdad and others (2004).

through the health care system is categorized as clinical preventive services; it includes such procedures as screening tests for cancer. Over time, a wide range of such services has developed. The U.S. Preventive Services Task Force, an independent scientific commission, reviews the evidence for clinical preventive services and makes recommendations as to its strength (Woolf and Atkins 2001), as does the Advisory Committee on Immunization Practices. In addition, the CDC-sponsored Community Guide provides updated, evidence-based recommendations on programs and policies to promote health at the population level.[2]

As with all medical research, some ambiguity exists regarding the effectiveness of preventive services and their application. Specialty societies sometimes disagree with the recommendations, and gaps exist in the research.

2. See Task Force for Community Preventive Services, "The Community Guide" (www.thecommunityguide.org/).

That said, prevention is unique among health services in having a decades-old, independent review group (the U.S. Preventive Services Task Force) that has spearheaded not just evidence reviews but also cross-service comparisons of services' impacts on health and costs. As a result, we have a good idea of what Americans and their health care system should be doing to promote health and wellness.

Low Use of Preventive Services

Despite clear health problems and known solutions, the U.S. health system has failed to promote prevention according to a number of measures. One way to assess this prevention gap is relative to scientific recommendations. One study found that only half of recommended clinical preventive services are provided to adults (McGlynn and others 2003). Only 38 percent of adults receive recommended colorectal cancer screening, according to the same study. The government reports that about 20 percent of children do not receive recommended immunizations, with higher rates in certain areas (for example, 41 percent in Birmingham, Alabama; see CDC 2006b). One of the major contributors to disease—high blood pressure—has become rampant: about 90 percent of middle-aged Americans will develop high blood pressure during their lives, although nearly 70 percent of those with this condition do not now control it (American Heart Association 2003). The statistics are similar for most recommended services. There are also differences in use by socioeconomic and demographic status: while 62 percent of non-Hispanic white seniors had received a pneumococcal immunization by 2005, only 32 percent of Hispanic seniors and 44 percent of African Americans had received it, despite having the same Medicare coverage.[3]

An alternative way to assess preventive service use is through international comparisons. In this regard, results for the United States are mixed. For certain services, like breast and cervical cancer screenings, the U.S. rates exceed those of other developed nations. However, only 49 percent of U.S. adults had their doctors provide them with advice or counseling on weight, nutrition, or exercise, compared to 72 percent in the United Kingdom.[4] The percent of elderly people who received an influenza vaccine

3. National Center for Health Statistics, "Early Release of Selected Estimates Based on Data from the 2007 National Health Interview Survey," figures 5-1 through 5-3 and data tables (www.cdc.gov/nchs/data/nhis/earlyrelease/200806_05.pdf).

4. Cathy Schoen and others, "Primary Health Care and Health System Performance: Adults' Experience in Five Countries," *Health Affairs,* web exclusive, October 28, 2004 (content.healthaffairs.org/cgi/reprint/hlthaff.w4.487v1.pdf).

Figure 8-4. Preventive Service Use and Potential Benefits[a]

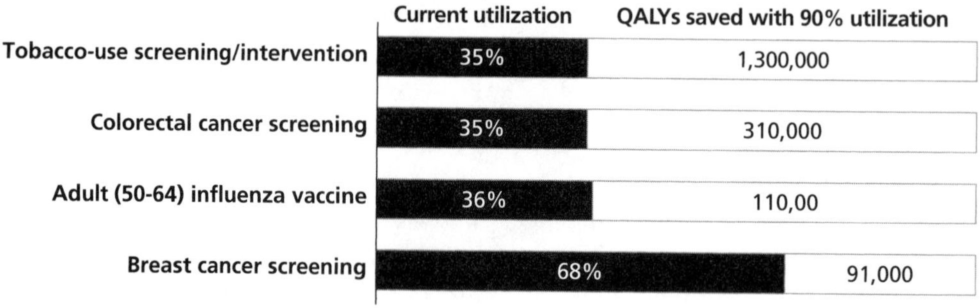

	Current utilization	QALYs saved with 90% utilization
Tobacco-use screening/intervention	35%	1,300,000
Colorectal cancer screening	35%	310,000
Adult (50-64) influenza vaccine	36%	110,00
Breast cancer screening	68%	91,000

Source: Maciosek and others (2006).

a. Utilization rates are for targeted populations. The current rate for influenza vaccines for seniors is 65 percent; the QALYs figure is for all people over age fifty.

in 2003 was 64.6 percent in the United States, well below Australia (79.1 percent) and the United Kingdom (71.0 percent), among others (Organization for Economic Cooperation and Development 2005).

Consequences of Low Use of Preventive Services

Low use of preventive services has a measurable impact on health. A comprehensive assessment found that three services—smoking-cessation counseling, aspirin to prevent heart attacks, and childhood immunizations—could substantially lower the clinical burden of disease (Maciosek and others 2006). If effective preventive services with low use rates were targeted, the achievement of 90 percent use could yield 1.7 million quality-adjusted life years (QALYs; see figure 8-4).

Similar results have been found for individual services. One study estimates that if effective risk reduction were implemented and sustained, the death rate due to cancer could drop by 29 percent by 2015, which would mean 60,000 fewer cancer deaths each year (Curry, Byers, and Hewitt 2003). Improved blood sugar control for people with diabetes could reduce the risk for eye disease, kidney disease, and nerve disease by 40 percent in people with type 1 or type 2 diabetes. Similarly, blood pressure control could reduce the risk for heart disease and stroke by 33 to 50 percent (CDC 2006a). A sustained, small reduction in blood pressure could reduce coronary heart disease by 21 percent, strokes by 37 percent, and cardiovascular death rates by 25 percent (He and Whelton 1999). A 10 percent reduction in serum cholesterol levels could reduce the incidence of heart attacks and strokes by about 30 percent (Cohen 1997). Studies have also documented that primary and preventive care can reduce the worsening of health problems that leads to hospitalization (Bindman and others 1995; Parchman and Culler 1994).

The health impact of the prevention gap has economic consequences as well. One study estimates that 78 percent of all health spending in the United States is attributable to chronic illness, much of which is preventable (Anderson and Horvath 2004). As the prevalence of chronic illness expands, so will its cost implications. For example, according to the CDC, the nation spent $174 billion on people with diabetes in 2007. The average cost per diabetic was more than five times higher than that of a person without diabetes. About 33 percent of the aggregate cost of diabetes results from work loss, disability, and premature death (CDC 2006a). Since the prevalence of chronic illness increases with age, its costs are disproportionately borne by Medicare. Between 1987 and 2002, the proportion of Medicare beneficiaries who were obese doubled while the share of Medicare spending spent on obese beneficiaries tripled.[5]

Prevention gaps also contribute to costs for acute illnesses. Preventable influenza presents a major cost to employers in terms of sick days and *presenteeism* (reduced productivity due to illness or other causes). Low rates of aspirin use after a heart attack contribute to subsequent heart attacks and costs. The failure to make prevention and primary care accessible also contributes to high rates of emergency room use for preventable problems. This not only contributes to the direct costs of delayed care through these settings but could also impose additional costs in terms of forgone health resulting from the lack of coverage. One study estimates that the societal loss associated with the uninsured in the United States ranges from $65 to $130 billion each year (Institute of Medicine [IOM] 2003b).

Barriers to Effective Prevention

The reasons preventive services are not used as recommended can be roughly categorized into four areas: barriers at the individual level, the

---

5. Kenneth E. Thorpe and David H. Howard, "The Rise in Spending among Medicare Beneficiaries: The Role of Chronic Disease Prevalence and Changes in Treatment Intensity," *Health Affairs*, web exclusive, August 22, 2006 (content.healthaffairs.org/cgi/content/abstract/25/5/w378).

structure of the health care delivery system, how prevention is financed, and limitations in public policy.

Barriers at the Individual Level

Lack of awareness of the value of prevention and specific recommended services is a major barrier to their widespread use. Generally, individuals neither know their own specific disease risk profile nor the preventive services they should receive. Nearly one in three people with hypertension, for example, is unaware of her or his condition (Hyman and Pavlik 2001). A similar problem exists among people with diabetes: about one in four of those with the disease does not know it, according to estimates. An additional 41 million adults have elevated blood sugar, putting them at risk for diabetes (CDC 2006a). The proliferation of information on the Internet could help raise awareness but has equal potential to create confusion about health matters (IOM 2004).

Even among those aware of the need for prevention, the attenuated relationship between actions and results diminishes the motivation to act. People have a limited ability to rationally calculate and compare the immediate time and monetary cost of prevention and the long-term benefits of additional healthy and productive years of life. Even when they appreciate its value, people may view prevention similarly to how they view retirement savings and do too little unless it is made easy and inexpensive. Moreover, some aspects of prevention involve challenging behavioral modifications and significant changes in lifestyle. The benefits may be too abstract to justify immediate and sometimes difficult actions.

Cost is a concern as well. It costs about $400 to $600 to fully immunize a child (IOM 2003a) and more than $1,000 for certain types of cancer screening. Without coverage, the cost of preventive services often constrains their use. For example, less than half—48 percent—of uninsured women ages fifty to sixty-four had mammograms in the past two years, compared with 75 percent of women in that age group who were insured all year. Only 18 percent of uninsured adults ages fifty to sixty-four had a colon cancer screening in the past five years, compared with 56 percent of adults in that age group who were insured all year (Collins and others 2006). Even some of those with insurance face financial barriers from either lack of coverage of prevention services or high cost sharing for them. Research suggests that cost sharing has a significant negative effect on the use of Pap smears, mammography, and counseling services (Solanki, Schauffler, and Miller 2000). Several employers, in designing their workers' health benefits, have found that eliminating cost sharing on preventive services improves use and workers' health without increasing costs (Busch and others 2006).[6] Nevertheless, neither public nor private insurers consistently lower cost sharing for preventive services as a way to encourage their use.

Ftn. 6

Structure of the Health Care Delivery System

Several aspects of the health care delivery system work against an effective wellness system. The first is its focus on curing existing disease rather than on preventing it in the first place. Most training for health care providers is geared toward making them action-oriented diagnosticians. They, along with their patients, often prefer therapies that provide immediate relief rather than screening and counseling that prevent problems perhaps decades later. One study found that among adults that had a doctor visit in the past year but who were not screened for colon cancer, only 6 percent were counseled about the test (Wee, McCarthy, and Phillips 2005). This is not surprising in a system designed around providing the sickest patients with the first and the most medical attention.

A second challenge is the nature of the health care workforce. Leadership within medicine has long recognized the importance of prevention and, to that end, has promoted specialties in prevention, family medicine, internal medicine, pediatrics, and gerontology. In addition, the number of physician assistants and nurse practitioners has grown. Nevertheless, the supply of providers who are trained to emphasize prevention is shrinking. Between 1997 and 2005, the number of medical school graduates entering family practice residencies dropped by 50 percent, from 2,340 to 1,132 (Bodenheimer 2006; see figure 8-5). Similarly, the percent of internal medicine residents intending to practice general medicine dropped from 54 to 27 percent between 1998 and 2003 (Garibaldi, Popkave, and Bylsma 2005). While the supply of nurse practitioners and physician assistants has grown, many of these professionals are being absorbed into tertiary instead of primary care. In the United States, relative to other countries, specialists account for a high proportion of visits and often act as primary care providers, despite their lack of the orientation toward prevention.[7]

A third challenge is time: delivering recommended preventive services is time consuming. One study estimates that it would take 1,773 hours per year, or 7.4 hours per work day, to deliver all of the U.S. Preventive Services

6. See Vanessa Fuhrmans, "A Radical Prescription," *Wall Street Journal,* May 10, 2004.

7. Barbara Starfield and others, "The Effects of Specialist Supply on Populations' Health: Assessing the Evidence," *Health Affairs,* web exclusive, March 15, 2005 (content. healthaffairs.org/cgi/content/abstract/hlthaff.w5.97v1).

Figure 8-5. Decline in Family Medicine Residents, 1994–2006[a]

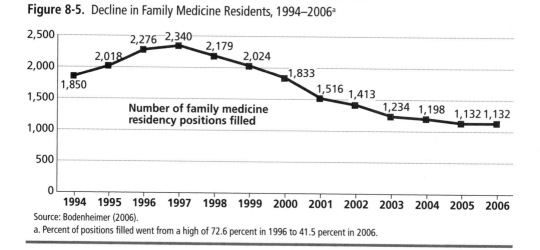

Source: Bodenheimer (2006).

a. Percent of positions filled went from a high of 72.6 percent in 1996 to 41.5 percent in 2006.

Task Force–recommended clinical prevention to a typical patient panel of 2,500 (Yarnall and others 2003). In addition, chronic illness management that comports to clinical guidelines would take from 3.5 to 10.6 hours per day, depending on whether the chronic illness is stable and managed or is uncontrolled (Ostbye and others 2005; see figure 8-6).[8] It would be a challenge even for a dedicated primary care physician to devote this amount of time to prevention.

There are also two aspects of prevention that differentiate it from other health services. First, there typically is no diagnosis involved; services are provided to groups of people who have no symptoms of disease. As a result, the decision about whether a service should be provided is made in advance and without clinical consultation. Second, there typically is no need for intense medical training to deliver preventive services. Some services such as sigmoidoscopies involve clinicians, but others require skills that can either be taught to nonclinicians (for example, injections) or are best provided by different types of professionals (such as alcohol abuse counseling). These characteristics present challenges in fitting prevention into the traditional medical model.

How Prevention Is Financed

One reason for the low emphasis on prevention in the United States is the nature of health care financing. Not only is there a lack of universal coverage

8. For a physician working forty-seven five-day weeks each year.

Figure 8-6. Time Cost of Prevention

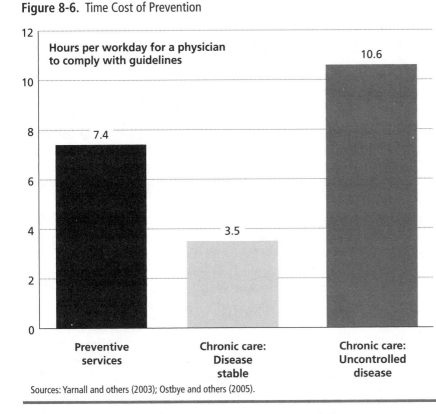

Sources: Yarnall and others (2003); Ostbye and others (2005).

in the United States, but few people—with the exception of those on Medicare—have the same health insurance plan for an extended period of time. The source and duration of health coverage depend on age, work status, marital status, and where one lives in some cases. Most Americans get health insurance as a fringe benefit through employment, which can exacerbate its discontinuities. A recent study found that the average person in his or her forties has already had eleven jobs.[9] Thus insurers have little incentive to invest in preventive services today that will benefit other insurers tomorrow (National Institute of Health Care Management 2003). This is especially true for those preventive services addressing chronic diseases

9. U.S. Bureau of Labor Statistics, "Number of Jobs Held, Labor Market Activity, and Earnings Growth among the Youngest Baby Boomers: Results from a Longitudinal Survey," August 25, 2006 (www.bls.gov/news.release/pdf/nlsoy.pdf).

that develop over a period of several years or decades, such as heart disease, hypertension, diabetes, and cancer. In these cases, the costs of prevention are incurred immediately when services are provided, but most of the benefits of reduced disease burden and avoided medical care are only realized in the future.

The lack of priority placed on prevention by insurers is apparent in both reimbursement and coverage policies. Pressure for clinical efficiency and productivity has compressed the average length of time available for physician-patient interaction during office visits. Quantity is generally valued more highly than quality in reimbursement. This makes it increasingly difficult for physicians to deliver all age-appropriate clinical preventive services, especially when they involve counseling, during a typical visit. One study found that high-volume primary care physicians were one-third less likely to schedule patients for well care and less likely to have high rates of preventive service use compared to low-volume primary care doctors (Zyzanski and others 1998). In addition, reimbursement for a diagnostic, surgical, or imaging procedure often pays three times as much as a thirty-minute patient visit that involves management and counseling (Bodenheimer 2006). Surgical specialists earn nearly twice as much, on average, as primary care physicians (Tu and Ginsburg 2006).

Insurers also do not uniformly cover preventive services. An employer survey found that only 64 percent of insurers cover cholesterol screening and only 16 percent cover weight-loss counseling (Bondi and others 2006; see figure 8-7). Focus groups with employers found that costs, employee turnover, and low use of such services accounted for their unwillingness

Figure 8-7. Insurance Coverage of Preventive Services, 2001

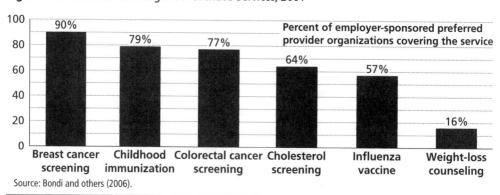

Source: Bondi and others (2006).

to cover prevention (Partnership for Prevention 2002a). Public health insurance programs also have gaps in coverage of prevention. Medicaid coverage of immunizations for influenza, pneumococcal disease, and other diseases varies across states, with two states failing to cover them at all for adults (Rosenbaum and others 2003). Medicare policy also has gaps: it fails to cover some recommended services (for example, screening for alcohol abuse), requires deductibles and cost sharing for others (such as colorectal and prostate cancer screening), and covers some services that are not recommended (for instance, an electrocardiogram in the "Welcome to Medicare" physical).

Limitations in Public Policy

Public policy could, and in some cases does, promote prevention. The system for identifying effective preventive services, described earlier, is government financed. Periodically, governments at the federal and state levels launch awareness campaigns (for example, National Breast Cancer Awareness Month). Demonstration projects in Medicaid and public health programs have added to the knowledge of what works with regard to prevention, and the public insurance programs have made some progress in covering prevention. For example, the U.S. Department of Defense has been a leader in incorporating prevention into its health system, recognizing its benefits for a prepared military.

However, there is no uniformity among federal health insurance programs and no national regulation of private coverage for preventive services—or most other health benefits. Health insurance regulation is largely in the states' purview. Some states ensure coverage of specific preventive benefits, such as breast cancer screening, but several of the recommended clinical preventive services are required by none of the states. Screenings for high cholesterol and blood pressure, for example, are required by fewer than five states (Partnership for Prevention 2002b). While experts suggest that national benefit mandates be considered for high-priority services such as immunizations (IOM 2003a), little progress has been made in moving this from theory into practice.

The public health system, as much as the medical system, is responsible for health promotion. State and local public health departments have a broad set of responsibilities, ranging from monitoring communities for infectious disease outbreaks to providing prenatal care. Nevertheless, despite repeated reports about the disarray of public health, few policies have been implemented to strengthen its systems (IOM 2002). Inadequate funding remains a concern. A recent report found that funding for public health is both unevenly distributed across states and insufficient, requiring an additional $2.6 billion to fill the shortfall (Levi and Juliano 2006). One study estimates that the CDC's National Breast and Cervical Cancer Early Detection Program serves only 15 percent of eligible women due to funding limits (Curry, Byers, and Hewitt 2003). In addition, a tension exists between supporting the often expensive delivery of clinical preventive services and using population-based interventions.

The Wellness Trust: Design and Rationale

The gravity of the problem of preventable disease, coupled with the inadequacy of the existing system, suggests that a new model is needed to prioritize wellness. To be effective, it should strive to make preventive services valued by individuals and providers available and affordable. It should elevate wellness within the health system and complement it with new delivery systems. Payment for prevention should be designed to leverage behavioral change and widespread use. Finally, it should be universal, providing recommended prevention services irrespective of individuals' insurance status.

A Wellness Trust is one approach for structuring an effective prevention system (Lambrew and Podesta 2006). Under this model, preventive services would be carved out of the health insurance system and financed through a new agency. The Wellness Trust would set national priorities for prevention, employ innovative and unconventional systems for delivering services, use payment policy to drive success, and integrate prevention with the health care system through information technology (see figure 8-8). The structure of the trust and its five major functions are described below.

Structure of the Trust

To concentrate and coordinate national wellness efforts, the trust could be established as an agency within the U.S. Department of Health and Human Services (DHHS), with a viable alternative being an independent agency. Its director would be nominated by the president and confirmed by the Senate. The term of the director would be at least four years, beyond any single presidential term. While the director would manage the trust, its trustees would make major policy decisions, similar to the process used by the Federal Reserve Board. The trustees would be chosen by the president, with Senate confirmation, from among the nation's foremost experts on disease prevention science, delivery, behavioral change, and financing, and possibly include key stakeholders. There would be a sufficient number to ensure

Figure 8-8. Structure of the Proposed Wellness Trust

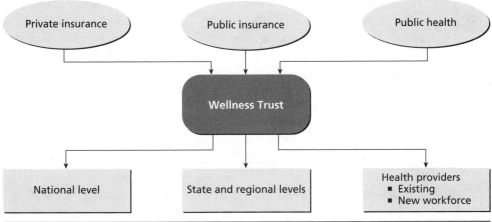

balanced decisionmaking, but not so many as to deter the development of a consensus. Decisions would be based on rigorously researched, scientifically based information and reflect a wide range of views, from those of consumers to those of specialists. This structure would allow for some immunity from changing political agendas and the pressures of special interest groups.

To maintain flexibility and agility in operating the system, the Wellness Trust would be given the authority to make decisions on specific delivery systems and payment methodologies. What the trust would do and how it would do it would be determined by the trustees; thus the ideas outlined in this chapter are intended to be illustrative only. The creation and functioning of such a trust would require a significant delegation of power from Congress and the administration. While daunting, the history of Medicare and other public health insurance programs suggests that delegation may be less challenging than creating, updating, and overhauling policies since, in many respects, being set in legislation is equivalent to being set in stone. Regardless, it would be part of the executive branch and subject to its rules as well as to congressional oversight.

The major decisions of the trustees would be issued in an annual report in which the trust would announce the prevention priorities for the coming one, five, and ten years and its plan for an effective delivery system for those priorities; present a description of its payment incentives; and announce the results of special studies it commissions. It would also release periodic reports and updates to ensure that the relevant information needed to guide the system is available. In the first several years of its operation, before assuming the role of primary payer of selected preventive services, its main job would be to commission and review studies to help it create the necessary infrastructure and decision support systems. Ideas for how this could work are described below. In practice, these policies would be established through regulation rather than legislation.

Function 1. Setting National Prevention Priorities

A major challenge in prevention is focusing on what works. Prevention can encompass a range of activities, from promoting smoke-free environments to undertaking highly clinical services to ensuring access to medications to control diabetes. The breadth of services is compounded by the emerging, multibillion-dollar wellness industry. The widespread use of some services may be less an indicator of what works than of what is convenient or popular. For example, the diet and weight-loss industry, which has few standards, is three times the size of the fitness industry, and both are significantly larger than the corporate or school-based wellness industries (TripleTree 2005).

The proposed system would begin by focusing on a subset of clinical preventive services that have strong evidence on their effectiveness. Unlike most areas in health care, prevention has an organization dedicated to reviewing its research. The recommendations of the U.S. Preventive Services Task Force, described earlier, have been widely used by providers and payers (Woolf and Atkins 2001). These recommendations would ground the nation's prevention priorities.[10] In addition, in 2006 the Partnership for Prevention sponsored a National Commission on Prevention Priorities that issued a report ranking preventive services on their health and cost effects (Maciosek and others 2006; see table 8-1). Such cost-effectiveness analysis is critical to determining the value of health care services and would play a major role in shaping the proposed prevention system.

Over time, the Wellness Trust would also consider for its list of priorities certain community-based preventive services. Such interventions, which are usually less medical and more behavioral, focus on populations rather than on individuals and are especially important to tackling obesity and tobacco use. The work done by the Healthy People 2010 project

---

10. Note that the Advisory Committee on Immunization Practices has the responsibility for developing recommendations for immunizations. This proposal assumes that this group would be folded into the U.S. Preventive Services Task Force.

Table 8-1. Prevention Priorities[a]

Units as indicated

Clinical prevention	QALYs saved	Cost per QALY saved (dollars)
Preventive aspirin use	360,000	None or reduces costs
Childhood immunization series	360,000	None or reduces costs
Tobacco-use screening and brief intervention	360,000	None or reduces costs
Colorectal cancer screening	185,000–300,000	0–14,000
Hypertension screening	360,000	14,000–35,000
Influenza vaccine	185,000–300,000	0–14,000
Pneumococcal vaccine	40,000–185,000	None or reduces costs
Problem-drinking screening and brief intervention	185,000–300,000	0–14,000
Adult vision screening	40,000–185,000	None or reduces costs
Cervical cancer screening	185,000–300,000	14,000–35,000
Cholesterol screening	360,000	35,000–165,000

Source: Maciosek and others (2006).
a. Ranked by cost-benefit ratio and effectiveness.

(DHHS 2000) and the CDC-sponsored Community Guide would be integrated into the new system.[11] Similarly, to the extent that there is overlap, the primary prevention focus of the Wellness Trust could be linked with secondary prevention (for example, chronic disease management).

Each year, the trust would determine and report on a list of prevention priorities to the president and Congress. Its trustees would review the recommendations from the U.S. Preventive Services Task Force and ensure that the list and its ranking reflect what is feasible as well as what is ideal. It is important to note that the evidence base for preventives services, like that of most health services, has gaps and gray areas. The trust would work with the research agencies across DHHS to develop and support the type of research necessary to determine priorities.

The proposed trust would use this prioritization in several ways. First, the list would be used to determine which preventive services should be financed by the trust. If financing for the trust is insufficient to cover all recommended preventive services, then the trust would limit its coverage to services with the highest priorities and allow the remaining services to be financed and delivered by the current system. The priorities would also be used in its communication function. Shifting emphasis from sickness to wellness involves more than just systems—it requires a change in culture.

11. See Task Force for Community Preventive Services, "The Community Guide" (www.thecommunityguide.org).

Having a clear goal, a priority list of services, and targets would help in the trust's effort to increase the value that Americans place on wellness. In addition, these priorities would guide payment policy. Incentives for individuals and providers would be developed around these priorities since their attainment would have the largest long-term rewards.

Function 2. Employing Effective Delivery Systems

This proposal would build systems around best practices in prevention, to allow form to follow function. One of the central functions of the Wellness Trust would be to match the prevention priorities with systems that would increase their use to 100 percent for targeted groups. It would do this in collaboration with the individuals and organizations that currently deliver preventive services, as well as with national and international experts. In the same way that its priorities would be based on evidence, so would its preferred modes of delivering them. While the trustees would determine the specific outline of the delivery system, some ideas for its shape are described here.

Preventive services can be roughly divided into three categories: immunizations and preventive medicine, screening tests, and counseling (Salinsky 2005). Immunizations and preventive medicine use biological material or chemical compounds to prevent the onset of a disease (for example, influenza vaccine or the use of aspirin to prevent heart attacks). Screening identifies risk factors or diseases in early stages, allowing for early and potentially successful intervention. Some of the screening tests are administered by physicians, involving invasive procedures or imaging technology (such as colonoscopy). Others require simple lab tests or exams (for instance cholesterol checks and vision screening). Finally, counseling consists of activities to try to change behaviors that are risk factors for diseases (for example, telephone "quit lines" for smokers). Despite their differences, these preventive services require the same conditions for effective delivery to their target populations: awareness of need by individuals and providers; accessible, affordable services; and catalysts to connect the two. The Wellness Trust would create these conditions through building infrastructure to support services, engaging and training a prevention workforce, and targeting state grant programs for health promotion (see table 8-2).

BUILDING INFRASTRUCTURE TO SUPPORT SERVICES. Infrastructure for a twenty-first-century prevention system would primarily consist of an information architecture. The trust would develop and implement an electronic prevention record system (described below under "Function 4")

Table 8-2. Prevention Delivery System

Service	Infrastructure for national priorities	Broadened prevention workforce	Restructured grants to states and regions
Immunizations and clinical prevention	Marketing, electronic health record, training[a]	Trained workers in schools, workplaces, pharmacies	Developing programs for children, seniors
Screening	Standards to improve quality Planning to ensure access and prevent overuse	Traditional health care providers for invasive procedures, imaging screening Trained workers in schools, workplaces, drugstores	Mobile technology Remote services
Counseling	National toll-free numbers National website for resources	Broad-based workforce including public health, mental health	Tailoring to vulnerable groups[a]

Source: Author.
a. These activities would be conducted for all types of services.

to ensure system connectivity, which is essential given its scope. In addition to identifying priorities, the trust would be responsible for providing information on them. It would maintain a central, up-to-date, accurate, and effective information dissemination system, including a website on preventive services. It could build on efforts such as Cancer Control P.L.A.N.E.T., which provides breadth and depth of information on cancer, options for prevention and control, and resources that are accessible in communities.[12] The trust would also operate toll-free telephone services with counselors for behavioral interventions such as smoking cessation. Experience suggests that highly trained operators on such quit lines have the motivational skills, time, and knowledge to effectively counsel individuals who prefer this type of contact (Woolf, Krist, and Rothemich 2006).

Another information-oriented activity of the trust would be a communications campaign about the importance of wellness. The trust would contract with social marketing experts to lay the groundwork for the shift in emphasis necessary to overcome inertia and barriers to engaging in health promotion and disease prevention. This is especially important in light of new evidence that social networks can have an effect on health-related behavior. In addition to direct marketing to the public, the trust could encourage promotion through wholesale distribution partners (for example, employers, school boards, local government, and food manufacturers),

12. See cancercontrolplanet.cancer.gov.

who in turn could affect retail distribution partners (such as work sites, schools, built environment, and retail outlets; see Maibach, Van Duyn, and Bloodgood 2006). It could also enhance the work of the new CDC National Center for Health Marketing, which helps federal, state, and local programs build in design features that improve their customer research, packaging, and distribution channels.

A more traditional infrastructure role for the trust would be workforce development. The Wellness Trust would coordinate training for a prevention workforce. New modules to train medical students and nurses would be created and implemented with the leverage of Medicare medical education funding, and new continuing education requirements would be implemented (Gebbie and Tilson 2006). In addition, the trust would train a new workforce to help run the proposed system. Certification programs would be developed around immunization, screening, and counseling, possibly as part of a broader effort to promote core competencies for public health professionals, community health workers, or both (Council on Linkages between Academia and Public Health Practice 2005; May, Kash, and Contreras 2005). Standards would be set and grants would be given to state and local educational organizations to provide this training. Certain groups of people would be targeted to become certified prevention health workers, such as pharmacists, school nurses, and human resources personnel in large businesses. In addition, the idea of training and recertifying a prevention workforce via the Internet would be explored.

In addition to the "software," or human capital, the trust would ensure an adequate supply of the "hardware" of prevention: imaging technology and immunizations, for example. Wide variation exists in both the price and quality of such services. To address this variation, some states such as Vermont and Connecticut have used a health planning process to prevent overuse and ensure adequate local access to technology such as imaging machines. The trust would consider assuming this role, since diffusion of technology as well as quality standards currently vary by state. Also, if it were paying for screening tests, the trust could competitively contract for such tests in urban areas, create loan funds to ensure access in underserved areas, and promote standards for excellence to limit false positives and retesting. This could reduce costs and improve quality in addition to ensuring access to preventive screening services. Similarly, the supply of certain vaccines has proven unstable. The trust would explore options for ensuring adequate supplies, including innovative purchasing arrangements or the promotion of a nonprofit drug industry (Pauly 2005; Hale, Woo, and Lipton 2005).

ENGAGING AND TRAINING A PREVENTION WORKFORCE. Most prevention supported by the trust would be delivered through its prevention workforce. Primary care physicians would continue to provide preventive services as part of the continuum of health care that is the hallmark of their profession. Generalists and specialists alike would be encouraged to provide opportunistic prevention as add-on services in acute-care visits. One study found a large percentage of elderly patients could receive recommended immunizations during chronic care visits (Nowalk, Zimmerman, and Feghali 2004). Physicians would also continue to be responsible for services such as cancer screening that require imaging and invasive tests. Similarly, the public health system has an infrastructure to deliver immunizations and community-based interventions; such an infrastructure is essential to the current and proposed systems.

However, new participants are needed to carry out the necessary functions to promote health beyond the traditional scope of medicine and public health. Many preventive services could be provided by trained individuals in sites more convenient to target populations, such as supermarkets, pharmacies, schools, and the workplace. Some of this exists today with the growth in retail-based health care centers that provide screenings, immunizations, and basic primary care. The workplace is also a growing and prime target for wellness activities. The proportion of workers with access to employer-sponsored wellness programs rose from 17 to 23 percent between 1999 and 2005, with a similar rise in the proportion who are offered discounts to fitness centers (9 to 13 percent).[13] Selected results are promising. For example, Union Pacific's aggressive antismoking counseling and medication program led to 29 percent of participants quitting smoking after six months (Leutzinger, Harter, and Craynor 2001). Finally, school-based wellness is critical since the trajectory of preventable diseases begins at an early age. The proposed system would train and help fund providers in all of these settings.

TARGETING THE STATE GRANT PROGRAMS FOR HEALTH PROMOTION. A third level of intervention supported by the Wellness Trust is regional and state grants. State and local governments have a long history of fostering effective, community-based health promotion programs. In this proposal, that role would continue, allowing top prevention priorities to be met with interventions targeted at difficult-to-reach populations through

---

13. See Eli Stoltzfus, "Emerging Benefits: Access to Health Promotion Benefits in the United States, Private Industry, 1999 to 2005," *Compensation and Working Conditions Online,* July 26, 2006 (www.bls.gov/opub/cwc/print/cm20060724ch01.htm).

community-based interventions. For example, the demonstrations from the Robert Wood Johnson Foundation's Turning Point Initiative suggest that locally designed initiatives that engage communities can be effective at changing obesity prevalence and reducing substance abuse in communities (Hann 2005). Group counseling, school-based activities, and mobile screening are examples of services that may be best organized at the state or local levels. Delaware's Screening for Life program, for example, provides educational activities in high-risk communities. Its activities include having health educators offer information at schools and churches and following those sessions with screenings in a state-owned mobile mammography van (Mitchell, Weiner, and Gage 2006). The trust would foster this level of intervention by working with the secretary of DHHS and the director of CDC to ensure that prevention priorities are reflected in existing grants. These grants would complement the work done by the trust at the national level and by the prevention workforce at the individual level.

This multilayered delivery system for prevention would be designed to maximize its cost-effectiveness. To that end, the best practices for an individual preventive service would be compared to those of other preventive, acute, chronic, and long-term care services to identify any overlap. For example, the infrastructure needed to promote primary prevention could also be used for chronic disease management, and vice versa (Woolf, Krist, and Rothemich 2006). Similarly, linking hypertension and diabetes screening could improve the latter's cost-effectiveness (Hoerger and others 2004). The trust would assess these potential overlaps as a way to reduce duplication of efforts and promote efficiency, integration, and simplicity in the system.

Each level of intervention would also be the subject of evaluation. The trust would work in collaboration with the CDC, the federal Agency for Healthcare Research and Quality, and other agencies that finance preventive services research and evaluation. Data monitoring and evaluation would be essential to determine whether a particular delivery system idea should be included or continued, as well as if it should be prioritized through financial incentives.

Function 3. Creating Incentive-Based Payment Policy

Under the proposed trust, a new set of payment policies would be developed for preventive services. These policies would aim to align the payment incentives with the nature of the service and ideal outcome. The trust's policies would be developed by its trustees. Ideas on how those policies could be structured, based on their level of intervention, are described below.

The national information services provided by the trust—such as social marketing campaigns—would be delivered through competitive contracts with private entities. Innovative marketing approaches that encourage millions of people to switch products could also help change behavior toward healthier lifestyles. Competitive contracting would also be used for some of the vaccines and imaging technology should the trust decide that efficiency and accessibility require that it take a greater role in their delivery. The use of competitive contracting would also limit the staff size of the trust and provide it with flexibility over time to redeploy resources toward different approaches.

At the provider level, the payment approach adopted would depend on the nature of the service. For immunizations and simple screenings, the goal is to encourage high volume in low-cost settings. As a result, payments could be linked to achievement of performance goals (for example, bonuses for immunizing a certain number of children or stepped payments that increase with volume). This would potentially improve quality as well since there is a well-documented relationship between volume and quality for services such as these.

A different type of incentive might be needed for complex screenings that occur in clinical settings. To convince busy providers to deliver such services, the payment for these preventive services needs to be on a par with payments for other comparable services. To ensure that their provision occurs and is of a high quality, performance incentives could be built into their payments, or prevention performance could be built into larger quality systems, as is typically the case today.

In the case of counseling, quality rather than quantity is the priority. It may take intensive counseling to affect a person's smoking, eating, or drinking habits. As a result, case-based reimbursement linked to outcomes might best ensure that services are available and effective. For example, certified individuals or organizations could be paid a fixed amount per person, with an upward adjustment for additional time only if it has been shown to yield a successful change in behavior. Proven performance over time would merit either higher annual rate increases or other incentives to sustain high performance.

These different approaches would share common features in the payment design. Within the incentive structure, each approach would have some base payment schedule, with adjustments for geographic price variation and different input costs based on existing payments for each service.

These payment levels could also be calibrated for the specific service's rank in the priority list. For example, bonuses could be given to providers for low-use but high-value services or for high-risk populations. Special attention would be given to payment systems for physicians to align incentives with optimal preventive service delivery methods and to balance rewards for prevention versus acute care and chronic care interventions. The typical concerns that a fee-for-service system may encourage overutilization would not be relevant in this case because the goal would be 100 percent utilization, and payments would be prohibited for more than the recommended usage or for provision to people other than those in the target group. The trust would not prohibit screenings or other interventions that are not on the priority list, but it would not pay for them. The trust would also consider contracting with managed care plans, public programs, or states for delivering prioritized preventive services if such programs demonstrate that doing so is cost effective.

The trust would piggyback on the Medicare payment system to transfer payments to prevention providers. Medicare already has relationships with the majority of health care providers in the United States. Through Medicare, the new trust would also pay the new, accredited prevention workforce and would reimburse Medicare for additional administrative costs. Medicare's payment rules and fiscal integrity systems would also apply. By having a centralized system and an electronic prevention record, the trust would ensure that no duplicative services are provided and that the first qualified person that administers a service is paid for it.

The trust would also use individual incentives to encourage take-up of preventive services. To facilitate the goal of full use of preventive services, there would be little to no cost sharing for those services with the highest value, as research suggests that cost sharing may be a barrier to use for many preventive services (Solanki, Schauffler, and Miller 2000). Other incentives would be explored as well. Some companies have implemented reward programs similar to those for frequent fliers to give people who use appropriate services a dividend. One hospital that gave employees $250 to $325 for meeting goals on prevention reported a 28 percent reduction in health care utilization during the first four years of its implementation.[14] The research on such incentives is sparse, but some suggest

---

14. See Wellness Councils of America, "Corporate Wellness Makes the Bottom-Line Difference: The Cost Benefit of Worksite Wellness" (www.welcoa.org/worksite_cost_benefit. html).

that short-term improvements in service use, such as immunizations, result from economic incentives (Agency for Healthcare Research and Quality 2004).

Function 4. Developing an Information Technology Backbone

The Wellness Trust would develop and implement an electronic prevention record. This would ideally be part of a larger electronic health record that runs the gamut of health care services. Short of this, an electronic prevention record would serve three purposes.

First, an electronic prevention record would provide a lifelong system for tracking the use of preventive service and would include the set of recommended services for each individual based on age, gender, and health history. This would ensure that no matter where or when an individual entered the system, a qualified provider could access information on what services that individual needed.

Second, an electronic prevention record would be used to promote wellness. At the provider level, the trust could build on the Electronic Prevention Services Selector recently launched by the DHHS. This tool allows providers to enter basic patient data to determine what services are recommended and access information for both providers and patients on actions to be taken.[15] Kaiser Permanente in Ohio, for example, uses computer-generated reminders to physicians to recommend aspirin for patients with heart disease; as a result, compliance has increased from 56 to 84 percent, with outcomes also improving (Kaiser Permanente 2000). Online tools have grown in popularity, and most major insurers offer them to members. This technology is also being integrated into coaching models, whereby individuals receive technology-enabled reminders, tracking, and other information to educate and motivate them.

Third, an electronic prevention record would be important for ensuring accountability and integration in a system that uses multiple settings. Since some preventive services would be delivered in nonclinical settings, an electronic prevention record would ensure that this distinct system is connected to both the medical and the public health systems. Physicians need to know whether a patient has received an influenza vaccine or mammogram; the public health system needs to know, for example, if

---

15. Agency for Healthcare Research and Quality, "AHRQ Launches Electronic Prevention Services Selector (ePSS) Tool for Primary Care Clinicians," press release, October 26, 2006 (www.ahrq.gov/news/press/pr2006/eppspr.htm).

there are geographic clusters of children who have low immunization rates; and the trust needs to know how financial incentives to encourage preventive service work and whether increasing such incentives has a corresponding effect (that is, whether there is a dose-response relationship). Since service use would also be noted in the record, duplication of services would be prevented. If linked to billing systems, this would also facilitate payment in multiple settings, and because the prevention workforce would be large, systems to protect medical privacy would be a priority. The development of such a record would be a significant undertaking, requiring interoperability standards, private protections, and full integration with other information technology efforts. However, such an electronic prevention record is the key to responsibly extending the boundaries of the health care system.

Function 5. Pooling Resources

The Wellness Trust would have a trust fund to finance priority prevention services. Spending from this trust fund would be considered mandatory, and it would have several sources of dedicated funding. Its authorizing legislation would create a methodology to carve out the prevention funding from Medicare, Medicaid, and other government programs, redirecting such federal funds to the trust fund. The trustees would assess what additional federal funding would be needed to eliminate underuse and to create initial infrastructure. Base-year amounts would be indexed by projected growth in national health expenditures in an effort to create parity with growth in spending on treatment of disease.

The trustees would also develop a methodology to accomplish a similar consolidation of private insurer spending. Because the trust would assume primary responsibility for high-priority prevention, it could create a tap on private insurers to help finance it (for example, dollar amount per person). This could be difficult to calculate and administer. Another idea would be to reduce the tax exclusion for employer-sponsored health insurance by an amount estimated to equal the trust's prevention spending per person with such insurance. Because the health benefits' tax exclusion value to individuals increases with their tax bracket, this would be a progressive financing method that would be relatively easy to administer. The estimated revenue from this change would be dedicated to the trust fund.

The general revenue dedicated to the Wellness Trust might also be designed to include some type of investment fund. In the same way that venture capitalists are able to pool up-front capital for investments that are likely to have dividends in the future, the trust could be given a small percent of funding to invest in services or infrastructure that could achieve long-term savings (Gostin, Bouffourd, and Martinez 2004). If successful, it would not only reduce costs, but it would also create a positive feedback loop for prevention investment.

No solid estimates exist on how much is currently being spent on prevention in the United States. This reflects two challenges relatively unique to prevention. The first challenge is that definitional boundaries are hard to draw (for example, identifying what component of a physician visit cost is associated with tobacco cessation counseling). The second challenge is that there are multiple sources of payment, including those that typically do not show up in the national health accounts. For example, firms' investments in workplace wellness range from $100 to $150 per employee per year, according to one report (TripleTree 2005). Spending on programs in churches, voluntary health organizations, and other nontraditional sites is also hard to capture. A 1992 study that thoroughly examined spending on preventive services, health promotion (activities influencing behavior), and health protection (changes in the social and physical environment) estimated that 3 percent of national health spending and 0.7 percent of GNP were spent on wellness activities in 1988 (Brown and others 1992). When these levels are compared with those of a much earlier period—1929 (see Falk, Rorem, and Ring 1933)—it appears that expenditures on wellness have only increased by 1.4 percentage points, despite the development of expensive screenings and early interventions, and the growth of the preventable disease burden. Furthermore, these levels of wellness spending are significantly less than the roughly 10–12 percent of health spending that occurs in the last year of life (Emanuel 1996).

Applying these percentages to projections for 2007 yields an estimated $70 billion of national health expenditures associated with prevention. Almost the same number is achieved by applying the original percent of GNP to the Congressional Budget Office's (CBO's) projected GDP for 2007 (excluding the amount attributable to health protection activities, little of which is counted in the national health accounts). If the proportion financed by public sources has remained the same, then the Wellness Trust might be able to capture $34 billion to $50 billion in public spending (at federal, state, and local levels; see figure 8-9). Note that this estimate is imprecise. A number of factors could make the spending higher or lower: the growth in the wellness industry, changes in underlying use patterns, differential price growth in prevention, and the nature and availability of

Figure 8-9. Rough Estimates of Spending on Disease Prevention, 2007

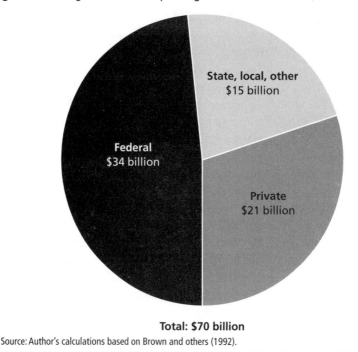

State, local, other
$15 billion

Federal
$34 billion

Private
$21 billion

Total: $70 billion
Source: Author's calculations based on Brown and others (1992).

other health services. This estimate is only intended to give a guess of what might be available for the trust fund.

Discussion

The new Wellness Trust outlined here would dramatically increase the nation's emphasis on disease prevention. It would both build on and compensate for the limitations of the current system for delivering preventive services. It would pool existing resources in an effort to redeploy them more effectively. Finally, it would strive to create a truly twenty-first-century infrastructure, where priorities, methods of delivering services, payment incentives, and feedback are based on evidence and information. The model is less like health insurance and more like public health or homeland security: it is needed by all people but not noticed if it works. That said, this proposal raises three major questions: will it fragment care, will it reduce health care spending, and how does it relate to other reform proposals?

Will It Fragment Care?

One could argue that taking prevention out of health insurance could fragment the system further. The problems of having multiple insurance systems can be seen in Medicare: employers, Medigap, and Medicaid all supplement it, creating complexity and administrative waste. This model moves away from the integrated "medical home" model that creates teams of physicians and other providers to care for patients (American College of Physicians 2006). It also could raise concerns from some health insurers who currently invest and innovate in preventive service delivery and want to keep that role.[16] Putting aside provider concerns, "blue sky" approaches typically entail transition costs. And because the trust would be new, it could acquire the politically damaging label of a big, new bureaucracy.

However, it can be argued that the existing health system has not done as well as it can in prevention, given the trends. From a sheer practical standpoint, the primary care system in the United States is at risk of failing to treat emergent and urgent care; it is hard to imagine significant expansion of its role in preventive care delivery without substantial changes in structures and incentives. The sharp decline in the supply of primary care doctors, coinciding with the baby boom generation's retirement, suggests that complementary systems must be developed. The same holds true for the public health system that has taken on the task of preparing for potential bioterrorism attacks and pandemics. Its capacity is already stretched thin. Moreover, the employer-based insurance system, through which most Americans are insured, is eroding. Fewer workers are covered, fewer health plans are integrated, and many plans have deductibles that apply to prevention as well as other health care services. It seems unlikely that we would be able to stop, let alone reverse, these trends.

The nature of preventive services also suggests consideration of a different paradigm. Prevention requires routine, population-wide interventions. Arguably, prevention is more analogous to public health and safety than to an insurable event. Preventive service provision is simple, repetitious, and often applied on a large scale across the population (Bar-Yam 2006). It also involves maintenance of health over time and across jobs. Information technology would provide the connective tissue needed to ensure integration of the prevention system with the health insurance and public health systems. An effective prevention system would also need to work with other social programs. For instance, school lunch and work-site health programs could be more important than medicine is in reducing obesity. With

16. They could keep this role under the proposal if it were cost effective to do so.

its outreach to new health workers and partners, the trust could achieve wellness better than a traditional, integrated health care model.

Finally, the Wellness Trust would sidestep two political impediments that might otherwise block effective prevention. The first is regulation. Rather than requiring private insurers and employers to finance and deliver prevention, it would pay directly for prevention. In so doing, it would simplify and prioritize services. This could be more acceptable across the political spectrum in an antiregulatory environment. Second, to be effective, a prevention system must operate in places where asymptomatic people go: work, schools, and shops. The ability to do so would be enhanced by the trust because it would engage private sector leaders in its own management and create a decisionmaking framework that is a step removed from the political process, with built-in inclusion of stakeholder input.

Will It Reduce Health Care Spending?

By definition, effective disease prevention and health promotion reduce sickness and delay death. Healthier or longer lives have prima facie value, irrespective of their net effect on health spending. There also appears to be a positive relationship between health promotion and worker productivity (Aldana 2001). An expanding literature focuses on the health benefits of services as measured in quality-adjusted life years and disability-adjusted life years. These measures capture both the extent to which services lengthen life and the quality of life in those additional years. Cost-effectiveness analysis aims to answer whether the potential health gained from these interventions is worth the marginal cost. Generally, an intervention is considered cost effective if the cost per additional QALY gained is between $50,000 and $100,000, although some experts suggest that this may be too low (see Ubel and others 2003). Though its methods continue to be refined, such analysis suggests that most prevention services meet this test. In fact, a broad look at the types of interventions that could improve the health of the elderly suggests that prevention stands out as having the potential to improve health and save money (Goldman and others 2006). The U.S. Preventive Services Task Force takes into account these types of measures when making its recommendations, as would the Wellness Trust.

While this information may be persuasive in allocating resources, policymakers typically want to know whether expanded use of prevention will produce savings in the health system. This is a higher test of cost-effectiveness whose result largely depends on the specific type of prevention's effect. To oversimplify, prevention that reduces illness without lengthening lives is more likely to produce budget savings than prevention that lengthens lives without reducing illness. Take, for example, tobacco use: increasing the use of screening and interventions from roughly 35 to 90 percent could save 1.3 million QALYs, more than three times that of breast and colorectal cancer screening combined (Maciosek and others 2006; see figure 8-4). However, these extended life years come with different types of health costs, offsetting potential health savings. In contrast, several interventions are so cost effective that they may actually reduce costs. One study estimates that if all elderly received pneumococcal vaccines, health costs could be reduced by nearly $1 billion per year (Hillestad and others 2005). Over twenty-five years, Medicare could save an estimated $890 billion from effective control of hypertension and $1 trillion from returning to levels of obesity observed in the 1980s (Goldman and others 2006). The potential for savings also depends on the effectiveness and targeting of the intervention. While their potential for improving health is great, cholesterol and obesity screening are at the low end of the cost-effectiveness scale for these reasons.

An even narrower question about savings is whether the CBO would attribute federal savings to a proposal such as the Wellness Trust. Here, additional variables get included in the equation. The CBO would assess what the potential impact would be on prevention utilization, how fast this would take effect, and whether, in the five- to ten-year budget window, any changes in utilization of other types of health services might occur (for instance, nursing home use could be reduced by effective reductions in high blood pressure and smoking; see Valiyeva and others 2006). It would also consider whether consolidation of funding and the payment systems devised by the trust would increase or reduce prices, what the administrative costs and savings might be, and how immune the trust would be from political pressure to fund priorities that are not evidence based. Last, the CBO would have to parse the costs or savings that would accrue to the federal government versus other payers in the system.

While it is complicated to address each of these questions, the premise of the trust (to redeploy prevention spending toward highly effective services) should result in some savings—maybe not initially but in the long run. Studies of similar, private sector interventions buttress this claim. A review of studies on such programs found that the return on investment is expected to average about three to one, although it takes several years to realize (Goetzel, Juday, and Ozminkowski 1999). A longitudinal study of one firm's wellness programs found a slight increase in costs for emergency room visits but decreases in mental health, outpatient, and inpatient care, for annual net savings of $225 per employee per year (Ozminkowski and others 2002). Finally, Freddie Mac, the nation's second-largest home loan financier, opened an on-site clinic at its headquarters, where 4,300 people work. It provides on-site preventive services, nutrition counseling, and routine care. Estimated savings due to increased productivity and fewer lost work days are $900,000 per year.[17] The Wellness Trust could also have other effects on spending. The trust would consolidate the administration of federal health programs' preventive services, eliminating the widely criticized stovepipe effect of the current structure of funding (IOM 2002). States would be relieved from enacting and enforcing benefit mandates on insurers to provide preventive services, such as colorectal screening coverage. Employers would benefit in two ways: lower premiums as prevention is implemented and, if it is successful, healthier and more productive workers. They could also choose to participate in providing prevention; if they did so, they would be reimbursed. For individuals, current financial, geographic, and time barriers would be removed. Given its mandated reliance on evidence, the trust would likely be more insulated from pressure to cover ineffective therapies (for example, fad diets). It could also limit inappropriate use of prevention (such as Pap smears for low-risk women). In short, while some costs would be associated with creating the trust and achieving its goal of increasing utilization of effective preventive services, the weight of evidence suggests that there could be net, systemwide savings.

How Does It Relate to Other Reform Proposals?

The idea of a Wellness Trust could complement both efforts to promote a patient-centered system and to expand health insurance coverage to all Americans. The proposed system has some elements in common with certain consumer-directed care models. Both place a high premium on information and on engaging individuals in their own health, and both consider financial incentives to be an effective tool in eliciting desired outcomes. The guiding principle of the Wellness Trust, however, is to make it as easy and simple as possible to connect individuals with effective delivery systems. In contrast, consumer-directed care plans generally expect individuals to take on more responsibility for organizing the system to meet their wellness, acute care, and chronic care needs. This is especially true with financing: rather than lowering cost sharing as a financial

17. Amy Joyce, "A Prescription for Workers' Health," *Washington Post,* October 9, 2006, p. D1.

incentive to use prevention at the point of service, many consumer-directed plans provide no insurance coverage for prevention, with 100 percent of the cost of those services coming from individuals' accounts, potentially discouraging use. As a result, the Wellness Trust may be more effective than consumer-driven models at incentivizing behavior that promotes wellness.

It also could fit within, and potentially accelerate movement toward, a comprehensive plan to provide quality health coverage to all Americans. The model could conform to any number of health reform plans, from a single-payer plan to an individual market approach that carves out prevention. A number of elements of the plan could also be enacted incrementally in the absence of major reform. For example, a cross-agency council could be created to improve prevention for people in federal health programs and thus lay the foundation for the trust. The development of a new health promotion workforce and payment system could begin immediately. Probably most important, an investment in research could be made to lessen the uncertainty around prevention priorities.

However, even if the Wellness Trust were enacted fully and immediately, it would still operate within a deeply flawed health care system. Uninsured people who were diagnosed with a disease through the Wellness Trust might not be able to afford its treatment. The high cost and relatively low quality of medical care faced by many will also persist without fundamental health reform. This is why the proposed wellness system should be part of a larger reform plan that ensures access to affordable coverage for all.

In closing, the Wellness Trust represents a major change in the organization and emphasis of preventive care in the United States. It would require new decisionmaking structures and systems for delivering and financing care. It would also require up-front spending, from both budgetary and political perspectives. Its potential to achieve its goals, like any proposal, is uncertain. Nevertheless, the cost of uncertainty may be smaller than that of the preventable health crisis that is emerging. The burden of preventable disease is escalating, and it will have broad-based implications for the nation, threatening to reverse the steady gains in life expectancy that the nation has experienced for a century. In light of such trends, the changes encompassed within the Wellness Trust proposal are critical.

References

Agency for Healthcare Research and Quality. 2004. *Economic Incentives for Preventive Care.* Evidence Report/Technology Assessment 101. Rockville, Md.

Aldana, Steven G. 2001. "Financial Impact of Health Promotion Programs: A Comprehensive Review of the Literature." *American Journal of Health Promotion* 15, no. 5: 296–320.

American College of Physicians. 2006. "The Advanced Medical Home: A Patient-Centered, Physician-Guided Model of Health Care." Policy monograph. Washington.

American Heart Association. 2003. *Heart Disease and Stroke Statistics—2003 Update*. Dallas, Tex.

Anderson, Gerard, and Jane Horvath. 2004. "The Growing Burden of Chronic Disease in America." *Public Health Reports* 119, no. 3: 263–70.

Bar-Yam, Yaneer. 2006. "Improving the Effectiveness of Health Care and Public Health: A Multiscale Complex System Analysis." *American Journal of Public Health* 96, no. 3: 459–66.

Bindman, Andrew B., and others. 1995. "Preventable Hospitalizations and Access to Health Care." *Journal of the American Medical Association* 274, no. 4: 1436–44.

Bodenheimer, Thomas. 2006. "Primary Care: Will It Survive?" *New England Journal of Medicine* 355, no. 9: 861–64.

Bondi, Maris A., and others. 2006. "Employer Coverage of Clinical Preventive Services in the United States." *American Journal of Health Promotion* 20, no. 3: 214–22.

Brown, R., and others. 1992. "Effectiveness in Disease and Injury Prevention Estimated National Spending on Prevention: United States, 1988." *Morbidity and Mortality Weekly* 41, no. 29: 529–31.

Busch, Susan H., and others. 2006. "Effects of a Cost-Sharing Exemption on Use of Preventive Services at One Large Employer." *Health Affairs* 25, no. 6: 1529–36.

Centers for Disease Control and Prevention (CDC). 1999. "Ten Great Public Health Achievements: 1900–1999." *Morbidity and Mortality Weekly Report* 48, no. 312: 241–43.

———. 2004a. "Health Effects of Cigarette Smoking." Factsheet. Atlanta, Ga.

———. 2004b. *The Burden of Chronic Diseases and Their Risk Factors*. Atlanta, Ga.

———. 2006a. *National Diabetes Fact Sheet*. Atlanta, Ga.

———. 2006b. "National, State, and Urban Area Vaccination Coverage among Children Aged 19–35 Months: United States, 2005." *Morbidity and Mortality Weekly Report* 55, no. 36: 988–93.

———. 2006c. "State-Specific Prevalence of Obesity among Adults: United States, 2005." *Morbidity and Mortality Weekly Report* 55, no. 36: 985–88.

Cohen, Jonathan D. 1997. "A Population-Based Approach to Cholesterol Control." *American Journal of Medicine* 102, no. 2A: 23–25.

Collins, Sara R., and others. 2006. "Gaps in Health Insurance: An All-American Problem." Report. New York: Commonwealth Fund (April).

Council on Linkages between Academia and Public Health Practice. 2005. *Core Competencies for Public Health Professionals*. Washington: Public Health Foundation and Health Resources and Services Administration.

Curry, Susan J., Tim Byers, and Maria Hewitt, eds. 2003. *Fulfilling the Potential of Cancer Prevention and Early Detection*. Washington: National Academies Press.

Emanuel, Ezekiel J. 1996. "Cost Savings at the End of Life: What Do the Data Show?" *Journal of the American Medical Association* 275, no. 24: 1907–14.

Falk, I. S., C. Rufus Rorem, and Martha D. Ring. 1933. *The Costs of Medical Care: A Summary of Investigations on the Economic Aspects of the Prevention and Care of Illness.* University of Chicago Press.

Fontaine, Kevin R., and others. 2003. "Years of Life Lost due to Obesity." *Journal of the American Medical Association* 289, no. 2: 187–93.

Garibaldi, Richard A., Carol Popkave, and Wayne Bylsma. 2005. "Career Plans for Trainees in Internal Medicine Residency Programs." *Academic Medicine* 80, no. 5: 507–12.

Gebbie, Kristine M., and Hugh H. Tilson. 2006. *The Human Dimension: Strengthening the Prevention Workforce.* Washington: Center for American Progress.

Goetzel, Ron Z., Timothy R. Juday, and Ronald J. Ozminkowski. 1999. "What's the ROI? A Systematic Review of Return-on-Investment Studies of Corporate Health and Productivity Management Initiatives." *AWHP's Worksite Health* 6, no. 3: 12–21.

Goldman, Dana P., and others. 2006. "The Value of Elderly Disease Prevention." *Forum for Health Economics & Policy* 9, no. 2: article 1 (www.bepress.com/fhep/biomedical_research/1/).

Gostin, Lawrence O., Jo Ivey Bouffourd, and Rose Marie Martinez. 2004. "The Future of the Public's Health: Vision, Values, and Strategies." *Health Affairs* 23, no. 4: 96–107.

Hale, Victoria G., Katherine Woo, and Helene Levens Lipton. 2005. "Oxymoron No More: The Potential of Non-Profit Drug Companies to Deliver on the Promise of Medications for a Developing World." *Health Affairs* 24, no. 4: 1057–63.

Hann, Neil E. 2005. "Transforming Public Health through Community Partnerships." *Preventing Chronic Disease: Public Health Research, Practice, and Policy* 2 (November): A03 (www.cdc.gov/pcd/issues/2005/nov/05_0072.htm).

He, Jiang, and Paul K. Whelton. 1999. "Elevated Systolic Blood Pressure and Risk of Cardiovascular and Renal Disease: Overview of Evidence from Observational Epidemiological Studies and Randomized Control Trials." *American Heart Journal* 138, no. 3 (part 2): 211–19.

Hillestad, Richard, and others. 2005. "Can Electronic Medical Record Systems Transform Health Care? Potential Health Benefits, Savings and Costs." *Health Affairs* 24, no. 5: 1103–17.

Hoerger, Thomas J., and others. 2004. "Screening for Type 2 Diabetes Mellitus: A Cost-Effectiveness Analysis." *Annals of Internal Medicine* 140, no. 9: 689–99.

Hyman, David J., and Valory N. Pavlik. 2001. "Characteristics of Patients with Uncontrolled Hypertension in the United States." *New England Journal of Medicine* 345, no. 7: 479–86.

Institute of Medicine (IOM). 2002. *The Future of the Public's Health in the 21st Century.* Washington: National Academy of Sciences.

———. 2003a. *Financing Vaccines in the 21st Century: Assuring Access and Availability.* Washington: National Academy of Sciences.

———. 2003b. *Hidden Costs, Value Lost: Uninsurance in America.* Washington: National Academy of Sciences.

———. 2004. *Health Literacy: A Prescription to End Confusion*. Washington: National Academy of Sciences.

Kaiser Family Foundation. 2005. *Medicare Chart Book, 2005*. Publication 7284. Menlo Park, Calif.

Kaiser Permanente. 2000. "Improvement of Cardiac Outcomes in Kaiser Permanente of Ohio." *Permanente Journal* 4, no. 2: 78–83.

Lambrew, Jeanne M., and John D. Podesta. 2006. *Promoting Prevention and Preempting Costs: A New Wellness Trust for the United States*. Washington: Center for American Progress.

Leutzinger, Joseph A., Chris Harter, and Bill Craynor. 2001. "Smoking Cessation for Blue-Collar Workers Using One-on-One Counseling and Bupropion HCl: A Pilot Study." *AWHP's Worksite Health* 7, no. 4: 33–39.

Levi, Jeffrey, and Chrissie Juliano. 2006. *Shortchanging America's Health, 2006: A State-by-State Look at How Public Health Dollars Are Being Spent*. Washington: Trust for America's Health.

Maciosek, Michael V., and others. 2006. "Priorities among Effective Clinical Preventive Services: Results of a Systematic Review and Analysis." *American Journal of Preventive Medicine* 31, no. 1: 52–61.

Maibach, Edward W., Mary Ann S. Van Duyn, and Bonny A. Bloodgood. 2006. "A Marketing Perspective on Disseminating Evidence-Based Approaches to Disease Prevention and Health Promotion." *Preventing Chronic Disease* 3, no. 3: A97.

May, Marlynn L., Bita Kash, and Ricardo Contreras. 2005. *Community Health Worker (CHW) Certification and Training: A National Survey of Regionally and State-Based Programs*. Report. College Station, Tex.: Southwest Rural Health Research Center.

McGlynn, Elizabeth A., and others. 2003. "The Quality of Health Care Delivered to Adults in the United States." *New England Journal of Medicine* 348, no. 26: 2635–45.

Mitchell, Nancy, Joshua Weiner, and Barbara Gage. 2006. *Case Studies of Health Promotion in the Aging Network: Division of Services for Aging and Adults with Physical Disabilities of Delaware*. Washington: Research Triangle Institute.

Mokdad, Ali H., and others. 2004. "Actual Causes of Death in the United States, 2000." *Journal of the American Medical Association* 291, no. 10: 1238–45.

National Institute of Health Care Management. 2003. *Accelerating the Adoption of Preventive Health Services*.

Nowalk, Mary Patricia, Richard K. Zimmerman, and Joyce Feghali. 2004. "Missed Opportunities for Adult Immunization in Diverse Primary Care Office Settings." *Vaccine* 22, no. 25–26: 3457–63.

Olshansky, S. Jay, and others. 2005. "A Potential Decline in Life Expectancy in the United States in the 21st Century." *New England Journal of Medicine* 352, no. 11: 1138–45.

Organization for Economic Cooperation and Development. 2005. *Health at a Glance: OECD Indicators 2005*. Paris.

Ostbye, Truls, and others. 2005. "Is There Time for Management of Chronic Diseases in Primary Care?" *Annals of Family Medicine* 3, no. 3: 209–14.

Ozminkowski, Ronald J., and others. 2002. "Long-Term Impact of Johnson & Johnson's Health and Wellness Program on Health Care Utilization and Expenditures." *Journal of Occupational and Environmental Medicine* 44, no. 1: 21–29.

Parchman, Michael L., and Steven Culler. 1994. "Primary Care Physicians and Avoidable Hospitalization." *Journal of Family Practice* 39, no. 2: 345–61.

Partnership for Prevention. 2002a. *Preventive Services: Helping Employers Expand Coverage.* Washington.

———. 2002b. *Preventive Services: Helping States Improve Mandates.* Washington.

Pauly, Mark. 2005. "Improving Vaccine Supply and Development: Who Needs What?" *Health Affairs* 24, no. 3: 680–89.

Rosenbaum, Sara, and others. 2003. *The Epidemiology of U.S. Immunization Law: Medicaid Coverage of Immunizations for Non-Institutionalized Adults.* George Washington University, Center for Health Services Research and Policy.

Salinsky, Eileen. 2005. "Clinical Preventive Services: When Is the Juice Worth the Squeeze?" Issue Brief 806.George Washington University, National Health Policy Forum.

Solanki, Geetesh, Helen H. Schauffler, and Leonard S. Miller. 2000. "The Direct and Indirect Effects of Cost-Sharing on the Use of Preventive Services." *Health Services Research* 34, no. 6: 1331–50.

TripleTree. 2005. *Health and Wellness: A TripleTree Industry Analysis.* Minneapolis.

Tu, Ha T., and Paul B. Ginsburg. 2006. *Losing Ground: Physician Income, 1995–2003.* Tracking Report 15. Washington: Center for Health Transformation.

Ubel, Peter A., and others. 2003. "What Is the Price of Life and Why Doesn't It Increase at the Rate of Inflation?" *Archives of Internal Medicine* 163, no. 14: 1637–41.

U.S. Department of Health and Human Services (DHHS). 2000. *Healthy People 2010,* 2nd ed. Vols. 1–2: *Understanding and Improving Health* and *Objectives for Improving Health.* Government Printing Office.

Valiyeva, Emira, and others. 2006. "Lifestyle-Related Risk Factors and Risk of Future Nursing Home Admission." *Archives of Internal Medicine* 166, no. 9: 985–90.

Wee, Christine C., Ellen P. McCarthy, and Russell S. Phillips. 2005. "Factors Associated with Colon Cancer Screening: The Role of Patient Factors and Physician Counseling." *Preventive Medicine* 41, no. 1: 23–29.

Woolf, Steven H., and David Atkins. 2001. "The Evolving Role of Prevention in Health Care: Contributions of the U.S. Preventive Services Task Force." *American Journal of Preventive Medicine* 20, no. 3s: 13–20.

Woolf, Steven H., Alex H. Krist, and Stephen F. Rothemich. 2006. *Joining Hands: Partnerships between Physicians and the Community in the Delivery of Prevention.* Washington: Center for American Progress.

Wu, Shin-Yi, and Anthony Green. 2000. *Projection of Chronic Illness Prevalence and Cost Inflation.* Santa Monica, Calif.: RAND.

Yarnall, Kimberly S. H., and others. 2003. "Primary Care: Is There Enough Time for Prevention?" *American Journal of Public Health* 93, no. 4: 635–41.

Zyzanski, Stephen, and others. 1998. "Trade-Offs in High-Volume Primary Care Practice." *Journal of Family Practice* 46, no. 5: 397–402.

Contributors

GERARD F. ANDERSON is professor of international health and of health policy and management at the Bloomberg School of Public Health, Johns Hopkins University; professor of medicine at Johns Hopkins University School of Medicine; director of the Johns Hopkins Center for Hospital Finance and Management; and codirector of the Johns Hopkins Program for Medical Technology and Practice Assessment. Anderson is currently conducting research on chronic conditions, comparative insurance systems in developing countries, medical education, health care payment reform, and technology diffusion. Before his arrival at Johns Hopkins, Anderson held various positions in the Office of the Secretary, U.S. Department of Health and Human Services.

STUART M. BUTLER is vice president for domestic and economic policy studies at the Heritage Foundation, where he plans and oversees research and publications on all domestic issues. He has written books and articles on a wide range of issues, including health care, welfare, privatization, and urban policy. In his twenty years with the Heritage Foundation, Butler has been widely recognized for his influence in shaping the policy debate and for his ability to work constructively with individuals of widely differing ideologies and backgrounds. In the fall of 2002, Butler was a fellow at the Institute of Politics at Harvard University. A native of Britain, he was educated at the University of St. Andrews in Scotland.

EZEKIEL J. EMANUEL is a breast oncologist and the chair of the department of bioethics at the National Institutes of Health Clinical Center. He received his M.Sc. in biochemistry from Oxford University, his M.D. from Harvard Medical School, and his Ph.D. in political philosophy from Harvard University. Emanuel has authored or edited seven books, including *Healthcare, Guaranteed: A Simple Secure Solution for America* and *The Oxford Textbook of Clinical Research Ethics*. His articles on the ethics of clinical research, health care reform, international research ethics, end-of-life care issues, euthanasia, the ethics of managed care, and the physician-patient relationship have appeared widely in the *New England Journal of Medicine, Lancet, JAMA,* and many other medical journals. Emanuel has been a visiting professor at UCLA and the University of Pittsburgh School of Medicine, as well as the Brin professor at Johns Hopkins Medical School and the Kovitz professor at Stanford Medical School.

RICHARD G. FRANK is the Margaret T. Morris professor of health economics at Harvard Medical School. He is also a research associate with the National Bureau of Economic Research. His primary focus is on the economics of health and mental health, with an ongoing interest in the organization and financing of care for people with mental disorders. He also studies economic policy issues related to the pharmaceutical industry. Frank received his Ph.D. in economics from Boston University.

VICTOR R. FUCHS is the Henry J. Kaiser Jr. professor of economics and of health research and policy, emeritus, at Stanford University where he is also a core faculty member of the Center for Health Policy and the Center for Primary Care and Outcomes Research. Fuchs uses economic theory to provide a framework for the collection and analysis of health care data. He has written extensively on the cost of medical care and on determinants of health, with an emphasis on the role of socioeconomic factors; his current research examines the inequality in length of life. Fuchs is a member of the Institute of Medicine and was president (1995) and distinguished fellow (1990) of the American Economic Association. He received a B.S. in business administration from New York University, and an M.A. and Ph.D. in economics from Columbia University. He is an honorary member of Alpha Omega Alpha Honor Medical Society.

JASON FURMAN is a senior fellow in the Economic Studies program (currently on leave) and was formerly director of The Hamilton Project at the Brookings Institution. Furman served in the Clinton administration as special assistant to the president for economic policy. Earlier in the administration, Furman was staff economist at the Council of Economic Advisers and a senior director at the National Economic Council. He also served as senior economic adviser to the chief economist at the World Bank. Furman has been a visiting lecturer at Columbia University, Yale University, and New York University's Wagner School of Public Service. He received his Ph.D. in economics from Harvard University.

JONATHAN GRUBER is professor of economics at the Massachusetts Institute of Technology, where he has taught since 1992. He is also director of the Program on Children at the National Bureau of Economic Research, where he is a research associate. He is coeditor of the *Journal of Public Economics* and associate editor of the *Journal of Health Economics*. Gruber received his B.S. in economics from MIT and his Ph.D. in economics from Harvard. During the 1997–98 academic year, Gruber was on leave as deputy assistant secretary for economic policy at the Treasury Department. He was elected to the Institute of Medicine in 2005. Gruber's research focuses on public finance and health economics. He has published more than 100 research articles, has edited four research volumes, and is the author of *Public Finance and Public Policy,* a leading undergraduate text.

JEANNE M. LAMBREW is associate professor of public affairs at the Lyndon B. Johnson School of Public Affairs, University of Texas at Austin. She specializes in health care policy and conducts research on the uninsured, Medicaid, Medicare, and long-term care. Lambrew is also a senior fellow at the Center for American Progress. Previously, she was an associate professor at the department of health policy at the George Washington University School of Public Health and Health Services. From 1997 to 2001, Lambrew worked on health policy at the White House as the program associate director for health at the Office of Management and Budget and as the senior health analyst at the National Economic Council. Lambrew received her M.A. and Ph.D. from the Department of Health Policy, School of Public Health at the University of North Carolina, Chapel Hill, and her B.A. degree from Amherst College.

JOSEPH P. NEWHOUSE is the John D. MacArthur professor of health policy and management at Harvard University, where he also heads the Interfaculty Initiative on Health Policy and chairs the Committee on Higher Degrees in Health Policy, which administers the PhD program in

Health Policy at Harvard. He edits the *Journal of Health Economics,* is a member of the editorial board of the *New England Journal of Medicine,* serves on the Comptroller General's Advisory Board and the Congressional Budget Office's Panel of Health Advisors, and has been a member and vice chair of the Medicare Payment Advisory Commission. He is a member of the Institute of Medicine and is a fellow of the American Academy of Arts and Sciences.

ROBERT E. RUBIN has been involved with financial markets and our nation's public policy debates all of his professional life. He began his career in finance at Goldman, Sachs & Company in New York City in 1966 and served as co-senior partner and co-chair from 1990 to 1992. Long active in both national and New York City's public affairs, he joined the Clinton administration in 1993 as assistant to the president for economic policy and as the first director of the National Economic Council. He served as the seventieth secretary of the Treasury from January 1995 until July 1999. Rubin joined Citigroup in 1999 where he currently serves as a director and senior counselor. He also serves as chairman of the board of the Local Initiatives Support Corporation, the nation's leading community development support organization, is a member of the board of trustees of Mount Sinai–NYU Health, and is a member of the Harvard Corporation. In June 2007 Rubin was named co-chair of the Council on Foreign Relations.

HUGH R. WATERS is a health economist and associate professor at the Bloomberg School of Public Health, Johns Hopkins University. His areas of expertise are health insurance and health financing reforms; evaluation of the effects of health financing mechanisms on access, equity, and quality; and economic evaluation of health care interventions. Waters has nineteen years of experience with public health programs and has worked extensively as a consultant with the World Bank, World Health Organization, and other international organizations. He holds a Ph.D. in public health economics from the Bloomberg School of Public Health and an M.S. in international economics from Georgetown University.

Index